I0838895

Dopey - A Journey to Freedom From Opiates

By Harl Adams

ISBN: 9798782226626
Imprint: Independently published

Dopey - A Journey to Freedom From Opiates

By Harl Adams

For Necia
my sweetheart for 51 years

About this booklet:

I hope this booklet will provide you the assurance that you are not alone in the battle to escape the world of opiates and that it will inspire you with the confidence to break free. Or that it will help you decide to never use them.

It is a very lonely place to be; in the company of a drug that may help you by treating your pain, but in the process it isolates you, makes you stupid, destroys your memory, takes you captive and binds you in fetters so tight it feels as if it will squeeze every modicum of life from your mind and body.

There are two battles to be won in this epic journey. First is the battle against the addiction to opiate drugs. Second, no matter how well one may fare in this battle with addiction, there remains the pain that initiated the use of the drug in the first place. If one cannot find natural painkillers (they do not work for everyone or for every kind of pain) one will still need their doctor to help them find prescription pain medication that does not take a person captive and put them back into bondage. Sometimes a person still needs prescription drugs but with the help of natural remedies the doctor-prescribed drugs may be effective at a lower dose. For some, there may also be the option of using an in-patient addiction treatment center.

If a person is taking an opiate for reasons other than physical pain, I believe, it is very important that that person also seek other help, other remedies. Non-physical pain is just as real as physical pain and there is help available to these persons to assist them in breaking out of the opiate prison. The US. Centers for Disease Control and Prevention reports deaths from drug overdose on a rolling 12-month manner rather than on a calendar year. As NBC news reports at https://www.nbcnews.com/health/health-news/yearly-drug-overdose-deaths-top-100000-first-time-rcna5656

"The number of overdose deaths rose 29 percent, from 78,056 from April 2019 to April 2020, to 100,306 in the following 12 months. The data, from the CDC's National Center for Health Statistics, is considered provisional but is a good indication of what the final numbers show next month."

"Deaths due to opioids – mostly synthetic opioids, including Fentanyl – accounted for more than 75% of the deaths."

If so inclined one can initiate a search for natural means of pain treatment. There are some excellent books in many libraries and available on Amazon. Some may want to know their options prior to breaking away from opiates.

This booklet is not a precision guide or a prescription on exactly how one can escape those bonds. It is written to show it can be done and what some of the obstacles one may face during their escape are. It is quite certain that one will have to modify these things to meet their personal needs.

Remember that licensed medical practitioners are the only people that can legally change prescription medications and/or doses. These same people may be able to prescribe medications that will help one to not have withdrawal symptoms or at least not have them so severely. The journey to freedom is not easy...or short; but it is worth it.

I desperately hope this booklet sparks a desire in someone to escape. If it does they should visit with a doctor and explore their options. A person may want to develop some distraction tools; make a schedule; identify friends that will help them, (don't forget pets) and trusted people who serve in addiction recovery programs and go for it! Reviewing the 12 steps of Alcoholic's Anonymous recovery program may be a good place for some to start; many thousands have begun successful recovery from addictions there. Those steps, along with links to associated material can be found at https://www.alcohol.org/alcoholics-anonymous/

Remember that the steps are not done one at a time.

Preface

The front part of this booklet provides some of my history with pain. This is not intended to spawn any kind of sympathy or make any "look at me" statements to the reader. It is intended to verify to the reader that my need for pain relief was great – remains great, maybe like yours, and I still had to go through the steps of finding out how my pain could be minimized (managed?) going forward without drugs.

Part of my medical history is included to show how desperate I was to find a treatment for severe pain that had gone on for more than a decade when I started taking morphine and three decades when I was completely clean. When I started using morphine it was only to treat pain. That never changed.

I realized I was addicted when I would get sick if I missed a dose of morphine and if I missed two I would begin withdrawals. This illustrates at least one of the risks of this drug. Another issue is the fact that many if not most persons who use morphine for long-term pain relief have to continually increase the dose in order to maintain the same level of relief.

I did not quit using morphine because my pain went away. My pain never went away, it only got worse. It got worse because my condition got worse and worse. I was on morphine for about 15 years. I had to learn or gain the belief that I could live without it.

My intent is to provide a frame of reference for the rest of the story... I hope it is helpful.

Dopey - A Journey to Freedom From Opiates

It all happened so very innocently so naturally, so perfectly, so logically, and yet it became completely consuming. I had never been the least bit interested in trying any drug recreationally. Except for treating migraines and injuries received in an automobile accident, it was odd thing for me to use prescription drugs for pain and I used fewer non-prescription drugs on a regular basis, even aspirin, Ibuprofen or Aceteminophen. I grew up in a home where we were taught the importance of not taking drugs unnecessarily and not taking illegal drugs at all. In fact we were taught that it was wrong to do so and I felt that was correct.

Automobile accident causes nerve damage -

In February 1992, just a few months after we moved to Maine, a fellow rear ended me at a stop sign which left me in terrible, unrelenting pain and nothing was easing the pain. The lingering pain required surgery. Several years after we moved to Texas, I had a nerve resection of my left occipital nerve (a section of nerve was removed by a neurosurgeon) in order to prevent the nerve damage in my back from registering terrible pain in my brain. That was mostly successful. However, there was and still remains near-constant pain across my left shoulder and down my left arm all the way to the ends of my left pinky finger and fourth finger on my left hand. Prior to the surgery I had been in pain that literally kept me awake nearly 24 hours of every day. In the five or six years between the accident and the nerve resection I slept less than three hours almost every night with only a few rare exceptions. Only complete exhaustion enabled me to sleep more than that on those rare occasions that I did sleep five or six hours. (Perhaps as many as four or five times a year.) I took no drugs for the pain during this time, beyond four injected nerve blocks. These helped but were effective for only about four weeks each. After the fourth block the anesthetist said that he would not do any more because recent studies indicated a possible risk of cancer with continued use. He said research suggested that more than three times may be somewhat risky.

Because of the pain and lack of sleep I had to spend tremendous energy focusing well enough to function, even at a compromised level. My work and to some extent some of my business associate relationships suffered. Family relationships were very disrupted, interfered with by the pain.

At that time we had several of our kids still living with us so I had plenty of company during the wee hours. The kids seemed determined to stay with me and not let me be alone in the overnight hours. I usually had one of them with me all night. During that time I decided on a distraction to help me to "keep my head in the right place". I wrote a book of 1,000 reasons I loved Necia (my wife) and had it printed for family members. I did write the full 1,000 reasons. Actually I titled the book *"One Thousand Reasons I Love You"* but wrote 1,001 reasons in an attempt to be cute. This took several years.

The kids would sit with me as I typed things into the computer. We had a nice time together. The only drawback was that I was nearly wild with pain; raw, grating on the nerves pain. Still, we would laugh and reminisce about experiences we had shared with their mother. We also relived some tender moments too. That distraction may have saved me. It also became my model for dealing with pain as time passed.

That was an education in pain. I figured that it should have lasted me a lifetime. It felt very much like most of the left side of my head was a tooth the dentist was drilling on with no deadening. That level of pain did not permanently diminish at all until the nerve resection. The pain was indeed a pain but spending time writing the book with three of our kids was a sweet experience.

Daily migraines triggered by pain from car accident -
I had my first migraine headache at the age of seventeen. Almost immediately after the accident they became a near-daily occurrence. A neurologist told me that the migraines were probably being triggered by the pain from the nerve damage received in the automobile accident even after the nerve resection. Other doctors concurred. The pain would have me vomiting and my vision would be so distorted that I could not read, drive or do other things that required focused vision. The pain would usually last several hours past the visual artifacts which is abnormal and actually contradicts the way migraines work. It took a great deal of effort to focus well enough to do just about anything. The first medication prescribed was just caffeine. I was not a consumer of any drink containing caffeine so swallowing a pill that was 100% caffeine was shocking to my body. It did not help the pain at all but after taking only one tablet I was very wide awake, and hurting, for nearly 36 hours straight! I didn't even get my usual 2-3 hours sleep per day.

The next migraine medication I tried was far more effective. It took a while to get to work but it would stop all but the most severe migraines if I could keep it in my stomach. This served me well for several years before losing its effectiveness. I felt fear and panic when it began to be ineffective because of the severity of my migraines. After several tries of different medications we discovered a medication that my migraine headaches responded well to. It was a new medication which has worked excellently for the last 29 years. It took one pill if I got it into my system soon enough that it would prevent me from puking everything up. If I did keep it down it would address the pain, nausea and visual artifacts within about 20 minutes...45-60 minutes if I had food in my stomach. It seemed like a Godsend. In about 2008 my doctor prescribed a medication that dissolved under the tongue which would prevent virtually all nausea and vomiting almost immediately so the migraine pill would stay in my stomach and be naturally absorbed by my body and perform its desired function.

Diagnosed with Paget's disease of the bone -

In 2002, multiple doctors diagnosed me with Paget's disease of the bone. The first pagetoid (tumor) set up residence in my skull and it hurt a lot! I may have had Paget's symptoms for several years prior to diagnosis but it intensified significantly by the end of 2002.

The first doctor to diagnose me with Paget's disease had ordered a standard blood test which included the measurement of alkaline phosphatase. That came back off the charts. It was flagged and the doctor had the test taken again to validate the results of the first test. The second test validated the first perfectly! That validation immediately brought on a serious discussion. I was informed that the levels were high enough that it meant one of three things, guaranteed: 1) I had liver cancer; 2) I had bone cancer; or 3) I had Paget's disease of the bone.

All other liver tests came back negative. All the cancer of the bone tests came back negative as. So, I was diagnosed with Paget's disease of the bone. A bone scan agreed with that and I was told that I had a Pagetoid in the right corner of my forehead just above and slightly behind my right eye. The doctors called the Pagetoid a tumor.

The word "tumor" was a panic word for me. I grew up in the down-winder area of the atomic testing done in Nevada. Although my family had none of the risk factors for cancer (smoking, asbestos, genetics, etc.) my mother, mother-in-law, and sister-in-law all died from cancer. All the males in my dad's family/generation had prostate cancer, one had kidney cancer. One of his sisters also died from cancer. In many ways the community seems almost like the people who survived the initial blast of the atomic bombs in Japan but died later from the effects of the radiation.

The certainty that there was no evidence of bone cancer was a great relief since several family members who died from cancer ended up in the end with bone cancer which had spread over most of their bodies, into most of their larger joints. They suffered much.

The doctor explained to me that even though the Pagetoid is a tumor it is not considered cancerous. (Although it can become cancerous; less than two percent.) No one knew how long I had had the disease. To this day no one knows what causes Paget's disease. The most recent bone scan shows that my brain was moving away from the pagetoid. My left optical nerve was sort of bunched up almost directly behind my left eye because my brain was right there. My right optical nerve was almost straight – just a little bit of a sag. It had to be to reach my brain. I am not certain I ever wanted to be normal more than at that time. Like a kid I thought I had had enough pain to fill my quota for a lifetime.

Like many other people who have a serious illness, I sought to understand why this was happening. I was thankful that I had my religious convictions to help me to understand that there is sometimes purpose in the things we suffer. Having a friend/companion like Necia was to have the best possible care – because she cared so much. Even when the pain made seconds seem like years, I felt blessed. Certainly I would never give up the pain if it meant I had to give her up also.

Incurable, can be deadly; little known about Paget's -

As I said, I was first diagnosed with Paget's disease of the bone in Maine. It was a bit on the frightening side to learn that I had an incurable disease that could kill me. Most of the doctors I saw for this disease knew very little about it. At that time I had two doctors tell me that their exposure to Paget's disease consisted of a single paragraph about one and one-half inches long on a double-column page in a medical school textbook. This is typical in my experience with this disease. I have seen two doctors who knew a little bit about it before they researched it in order to work with me. I do not say this to be critical; it was just how it was. One of the doctors at the University of Utah who several of my other doctors referred to as the expert on Paget's disease put it into perspective for me, "This disease is so rare and such a small part of those who do get it are ever symptomatic that there are no studies done because almost nobody knows anyone with the disease who has symptoms, so, no one funds research and until something causes the pharmaceutical companies to think there is a great opportunity for them; they aren't interested." "The only other possibility is for some extremely wealthy person to get the disease and fund a study. However if a wealthy person did fund *a* study...that would be exactly one study. Many studies may be necessary in order to find a treatment that is effective."

Few who have Paget's disease have pain; those who have pain, have severe pain -

When I was diagnosed with Paget's disease of the bone some doctors and most internet sites were still claiming that this was not a painful disease. However, within a couple of years following my diagnosis that began to change. Now some doctors call it a disease of agony for the small percentage of people who are symptomatic. Most people who have Paget's disease of the bone do not know they have it until it is noticed while the doctor is looking for something else, usually using the alkaline phosphatase test or they have twisting of one or more of the long bones in their body or excessive bone growth in their skull. In most cases their skull grows outward. In my case the growth in my skull is inward. One doctor in Boston said that, "when someone with symptomatic

Paget's enters a room they usually lead with their head." Suggesting that the bone growth, which is usually on the outside of the skull, makes one's head obviously larger than normal.

One day, quite a while after I had been diagnosed, I said to my doctor, "I know that this disease is not supposed to be painful so I must have quite an imagination because my head hurts terribly all of the time; sometimes it is unbearable." The doctor asked us, my wife, Necia and I, to wait while he verified something. He left the room for about 20 minutes, when he returned he told us that Paget's disease of the bone was *nearly always* asymptomatic. However, those few who do have pain, have severe pain. He had consulted the latest materials Intermountain Health Care (IHC) provided their doctors. I have found myself wishing, many times, that it had just been my imagination.

Today it is possible to see and feel (with my fingers) where the changes in the bone has caused a bit of disfigurement on both sides of my forehead. (And I can certainly feel the pain!) It might look a little worse but since I never considered myself to be a "looker" it has not bothered me. The pain *HAS* bothered me. It would look considerably different if my growth were on the outside of my skull. It is also likely that I would not have so many other symptoms that were not easily explained. Mostly neurological.

One of the new things about Paget's was that if I bend over or do something that makes me strain – perhaps lifting a heavy object, the increase of pressure in my head often sets off severe pain...more than the severe that is there virtually all of the time. Cold also sets off the pain. I wear a beanie cap when I am in church. People have been very kind and tolerating...we are all thinking that the Lord knows what is going on and he is okay with it as long as it is needed. Pretty goofy looking but as long as it is winter or the air conditioner is running I must have some kind of cap on no matter where I am. The cap must be warm and cover the places where the Paget's is active in my head. This now means much of my head. In 2020 a neurologist studying the latest MRI of my head pointed to a white band which extended all of the way around my skull and told us that that was all Paget's-related bone growth.

Many times I have played the part of the vain person as I have stood and looked into a mirror for long minutes trying to see what was making me hurt so much. It seems nearly impossible that something which hurts so much cannot be seen from a long way off. Not so in my case.

Disease spreads, more of the inside of my skull affected -
The pain continued to increase in intensity and became omnipresent; it hurt all the time. The silver lining to this cloud was that it did not hurt at the highest intensity all of the time. I was reminded that there was no cure and no treatment for the disease and people did not recover from it on their own. In short, I had this disease for life. And yes, Paget's disease would or could be what

finally ended a few people's lives; mine included. More doctors agreed that the pain caused by Paget's disease was now triggering the increased daily migraines. So even though the worst of the car-wreck pain was addressed with the nerve resection, Paget's had taken over in triggering terrible daily migraines.

Some doctors had begun to prescribe the same medicine for Paget's disease of the bone that was prescribed for people with severe osteoporosis. I took one of those medicines for several years at a dose that was more than seven times the typical dose given to patients with osteoporosis. It was costing us about $1,000 monthly for this medication alone. This and other medications took a pretty large bite out of our retirement savings. At one point I was taking four medications for pain. I felt that I should own stock in a pharmaceutical company; perhaps in all of them.

When Paget's disease hurts it hurts a lot and it kills people-

One source that Necia read, said that people with symptomatic Paget's disease of the bone could expect to live an average of five years after becoming symptomatic. That was spooky but after a while it just faded into the collage that was my medical records. At this writing I have lived 19 years, nearly a third of my life at this point, since diagnosis and onset of symptoms.

Along with the pain were feelings of a general state of sickness. Whenever the pain was bad I could expect to feel terribly sick almost right away. Sometimes the pain caused me to throw up. I tried to make a joke that Paget's disease was sickening. That has never changed. As the pain increased so did the severity of the sickness and sometimes also the intensity of my puking. There were, at times, great fits of puking caused by migraine headaches whenever I failed to get the anti-puke medicine and the new migraine medicine into my body soon enough. Sometimes my retching would bring up bile and blood. When Paget's and a migraine party together I am rendered brain-dead-stupid. I struggle to make sense of just about anything. Thankfully I can stop most migraines in their tracks.

So, more significant, more painful, more consuming than the damage from the car wreck and the migraines it triggered was the Paget's pain and the almost daily migraines now triggered by Paget's. How could a disease I had never heard of be so painful? Again I say thanks for the effective migraine treatment.

No effective treatment – anywhere -

I saw more than 45 doctors for this problem (Paget's and the associated pain and neurological symptoms) in Maine Medical Center, Southern Maine Medical Center, Maine Neurology, University of Vermont, Massachusetts General Hospital, University of New England, Snow Canyon Clinic (neurology), Intermountain Health Care St. George Hospital, and the University of Utah, as well as numerous other specialists/clinics. As I said earlier, I was prescribed one of the medications given to people who have serious osteoporosis. I felt no change when I took this medicine, the pain continued to be severe. I thought the medication was to slow the spread and advancement of the Paget's growth. Finally I saw a doctor at the University of Utah (one who was referred to as *THE* expert in Utah) who advised me that the only reason they prescribed that medication to people with active Paget's was an attempt to relieve some of the pain. To ensure that I was not making a poor decision to stop taking it the doctor had me run a test of not taking the medication for two weeks and noting the pain severity, then taking it for two weeks and comparing the results. The medication was doing me no good. Nothing helped the pain.

By the time I had been symptomatic for a couple of years I was pretty well consumed with pain. I did not have to have some external thing remind me that I was hurting. I found myself, almost naturally, deliberately trying to focus my thoughts away from the pain. I had arrived at a point when I had to do this in order to survive. The pain was severe, debilitating. It affected, perhaps controlled my mood, and I found myself saying stupid, cruel, senseless things without a clue why. I had no idea where those thoughts and words came from. I still cannot explain it. It remained that bad and on many days worse. I had to have some help with the pain. I could not do this any longer; I really needed medicine. Help!

Around this time we were excited to learn that a rheumatologist was starting a practice about 50 miles away. These are the doctors who work on diseases that affect joints tendons, ligaments, bones, and muscles. Thus Paget's disease ends up in their domain. We called and made the earliest appointment available which was for about six months out. A couple of weeks before the appointment date his office called and asked me why I needed to see him. When I responded with "Paget's Disease of the Bone" they then informed me that he did not accept patients with Paget's of the bone. That was extremely discouraging; one more doctor confirming that he could do nothing. And he was an "expert". That did save $$$ for us.

Pain was severe and yet I could sleep 12 hours on just about any given day; other days I could not sleep at all –

I had several symptoms which really caused considerable frustration for the doctors and I. One of those symptoms was the fact that sometimes I could not sleep at all because of the pain and much of the time I had to have *at least* 12 hours of sleep in order to function at all. Several symptoms were considered neurological but after the Paget's had progressed somewhat most doctors said the other symptoms were artifacts of the bone growth inside my skull and the resulting affect on my brain. At about this time I thought I would be cute and just say that my problems were all in my head. I said that to many doctors and they mostly smiled and said nothing. One laughed heartily.

But everything was about to change...

Started taking morphine which reduced the level of pain - but not always, never completely eliminated the pain -

During this same period of time my primary care doctor referred me to <u>another</u> neurologist who reminded me that there was no standard treatment for the pain associated with Paget's disease. I told him I needed some relief. He quizzed Necia and I about my history, what I had taken, how much, for how long, did it help... Satisfied that I was not just shopping for drugs he prescribed morphine. His immediate predecessor had run a complete workup on scans and lab work so he also had that information to show there was a reason for my pain. During this time I had three 'spinal taps' (lumbar punctures) as the doctors kept searching for other illnesses. Those in the autoimmune group seemed what most of them suspected. Unfortunately I have Paget's Disease; fortunately I have not been found to have an autoimmune disease.

I hate to hurt. I truly HATE to hurt. Even so, I quickly learned to hate morphine but it usually relieved the pain enough that I was grateful to have the morphine available. I was dopey but hurting on this scale was eased some for a few years.

This doctor had a pretty good sense of humor. When he handed me the first prescription for morphine he said, "now I want you to remember that the dog can eat your homework only once, do you understand what I am saying"? I was a bit slow on that day so he said it straight up, "If you happen to lose a prescription or lose your pills I will give you a new prescription but that cannot ever happen a second time because I will never do that again no matter what reason you may have". I understood clearly and was terrified.

People judge; Doctors told me I must leave the workforce -

Everyone seems to have different coping mechanisms for different problems. There were also a couple of things I learned to resent: 1) I really resented it when people would say things like "well, you don't look like you are hurting very much to me"; and 2) When they wanted to grill me to hear every detail of what the doctors were telling me and then attempt to help me out and re-diagnose my illness. If anyone were to know how hard I worked to hide the fact that I was hurting because I did not want to be the focal point of any discussion, they could not possibly believe what they were saying. But, I bitterly resented anyone who told me I was not feeling any pain and was just wanting to not have to work anymore or I just needed to "suck it up". I did not want to have such a discussion with anyone because almost all I cared about was not hurting and did not want to justify taking medication, legally prescribed and taken per the prescription, to anyone. Beside that, is the fact that I enjoyed my job and *liked* to work. I had a great job and it broke my heart to have to leave it.

Perhaps as you read this you will be able to find common experience with me. Don't most people feel stupid or at least silly trying to convince someone they are not some selfish knave. Sometimes people would make jokes about how they wished they could take large doses of opioid medication. These were sometimes the same people who condemned me for taking it. When a fellow hurts so badly that even the simplest of verbal exchanges is sometimes very hard work it is not easy to take the criticism or judgment or, as some may put it the accusations. Again, when the doctors told me I needed to leave the workforce, it was a terrible blow to me.

Began using distraction to help cope with pain -
I was a goof-off. That is how I dealt with 'hiding' pain. I had to be busy, focused and yet distracted from the pain. Distracted is a word that describes it best. I figured that since I could not control the pain I had to find a way of living with it. Goofing off and trying to be funny, clever... anything that would distract me enough to push through the pain was justified in my mind. For several years those same behaviors seemed to work most of the time in deflecting the attention given. I admit that I am not very funny.

Sometimes it was essential to have some predetermined distractions which are only mental. When possible it is nice to have something you can do that is physical. Of course "physical" may often increase the level of pain. Clearly, it is not an effective distraction if it elevates the level of pain. (Duh!) This last sentence is obvious but necessary; especially in the context where a certain type of physical activity may effectively distract one's attention away from the pain for a short period of time but leave one in increased pain for a longer time going forward. I had multiple misfires on this type of distraction. Indeed I paid "the Piper" more than a few times for this behavior. I now call it a destructive behavior vs a distracting behavior.

It is nice to have friends that love you. It is nice to have people you respect and care about to empathize with you. My best friends cared about how I was doing but never made jokes, accused or attempted to re-diagnose me. They were also very earnest in their understanding and desire for me to not continue to hurt or to hurt at an increased level. My family has been the same; they fully understand that I sometimes had to decide at the last minute that I could not do something – even something that was special and had been planned for some time. Frustratingly, this was caused as often by the morphine as it was by the pain. Morphine is a disabling drug.

Pain was severe; kidney stones not nearly as bad even before I began to take morphine -

It helped my family understand my pain as they watched me pass numerous kidney stones with no pain medication. The truth is that my head usually hurt much worse than the kidney stones. It would rattle my doctors when I produced some kidney stones from my pocket and they would ask me what hospital I went to or what drugs I had taken and finally why didn't I call them? One of them got very rude and made fun, accused me of trying to be "some kind of a Superman". Nope. It was just that my head hurt so much more than the kidney stones that the stones were a v-e-r-y secondary concern. I must admit, however, that kidney stones do hurt!

Perhaps others who are taking strong drugs for pain have also been judged for doing so. I have not usually worried too much about what others thought of the decisions I made in living my life. But for some reason, hearing the false accusations, the attempted jokes and the constant attention some people gave the fact that I was taking hefty doses of morphine did get under my skin. I would just avoid people who gave me a difficult time. I don't know how most people even knew I was taking morphine.

I must add the fact that there are many kind, caring people who tried to understand and were non-judgmental and actually tried to not treat me differently except when some fact was in the way such as when someone wanted people to assist in driving kids in a church youth group someplace. The fact that I could not drive and take this much medication was readily accepted by most. Many kind people just acknowledged the situation and moved on with what they were doing without making me some kind of spectacle or villainizing me. Most people did wish me well when this kind of thing happened.

I found myself being somewhat of a hypocrite. As much as I sometimes resented others making jokes at my expense, I would make jokes about my life. I have probably used a line like, "Don't worry about me, all my problems are in my head" a hundred times. I don't know why I would do and say what I did but then resented it so much when others tried to joke about it. Perhaps this is one way through which it became known, by some, I was a user of morphine.

The neurologist who first prescribed morphine to treat my pain seemed to be very concerned, disciplined, serious and methodical in his prescription of morphine. He started me out on a very low dose and gradually increased it until the pain was partially treated. We agreed that I did not want to take more than enough to keep my pain only at a livable level. I figured I would be doped completely silly, perhaps comatose, if I took enough to make all of the pain go away and I hate how it feels to be dopey. And morphine does make me dopey, goofy. Not the Disney characters of Dopey and Goofy; no, much worse. It is a fact that I began to lose function long before the morphine addressed the pain to any level that gave me function. However, at first that seemed like a reasonable trade-off because it was such a relief to have at least a part of the pain abated. By the time any significant pain reduction was realized I had lost a great deal of my memory function, my brain function in general was seriously compromised, my ability to reason and make decisions was extensively affected. It did not take me long to begin avoiding making decisions...and/or I would just rattle off a decision that was the first thought that came into my mind. I frustrated some who were close to me with this obviously cavalier behavior. It was obvious when I made these "snap" decisions that most of them were foolish, unreasonable, stupid, reckless, etc. But the decisions were made, done, finished, and I did not have to worry about them – until the consequences of the decisions arrived. Yes, even though the consequences did come, as the doses of morphine increased so did my unreasoned decision-making.

The most glaring painful consequence of this decision avoidance and the choice I made to just go with the first thing that entered my mind was that I would just say that first thing that came to my mind. I said many, many really stupid things. Some were hurtful, many were just foolish/stupid; only on the rare occasion were my decisions wise. I qualified completely as dopey. And in every instance more morphine meant more dopey. I hated myself for saying stupid or cruel things but at the same time I continued to be irresponsible just because it was so difficult to make my mind focus and think. I was often in the mode of "just say it and move on". This did not make me good company. This did not make me happy. Quite the contrary, it made me unhappy and added to the burdens produced by this mind-numbing, mind-bending drug. More dopey.

Morphine is not all created equal; pain management difficult -
To begin with the neurologist prescribed a morphine which was supposed to be the Cadillac brand. A person was supposed to be able to take it in twelve-hour or twenty four hour doses. My system did not like that dosing since my body consistently used up (some said "metabolized) the twelve-hour dose in ten hours. The 24-hour dose was similarly affected. Thus, I had good pain management for ten or 20 hours; after that I was a mess for two (or four) hours plus however much time it took for the morphine to start working after I took the next dose. That sometimes took several days for my body to level out again. We tried to play games with different mixtures of extended release and immediate release options but could not get things right so we just relied on extended release for everything except breakthrough pain, for several years. We used immediate release for break-through pain. Later on we added immediate release to each dose to prevent me losing pain control when the level got too low at the dosing time. At this same time we switched to a generic extended release morphine which worked much better. We also switched to dosing three times per day vs the previous dosing of two times per day. Even dosing three times per day changing to the generic saved us hundreds of dollars each month. (Hitting our retirement savings.)

I never got comfortable on morphine; I resented everything about what it did to me except take away physical pain. In those days avoiding physical pain was my passion. I remain pain-averse but I remain even more resentful about all the side effects of morphine.

I always liked being outside. I have always thought this world to be a beautiful place. I have pretended to write poetry which declared this fact many times. A couple of times it even turned out at least mediocre. However, morphine dimmed the stars, took the fresh smell from the flowers and made the animals in nature all look less pretty. It robbed me of nearly everything that is naturally beautiful. Sure, all that stuff was still there but it was boring...sometimes irritating. Figure out the logic of that!

It is very difficult to re-establish effective pain management when control is lost. Whenever my body "metabolized" the medication hours prior to my next dosing, it did not just cost me two hours of pain. It also took time for the next dose to take effect and that does not occur very readily. I needed a dosing schedule and a cooperating medicine so that I did not ever lose control. The generic morphine sulfate extended release on an eight-hour dosing schedule was the solution.

In the long run I could get better treatment of my pain on a lower dose of morphine if I could maintain control. This may not make sense to a person who has not been a part of this business of pain management. This caused me a lot of frustration over the years. I began to carry one full dose and several extra immediate release tablets, for break-through pain, with me at all times. This began after we had gone some place and been delayed long enough to miss a couple of doses.

If I were to become someone's 'advisor' (I never want to) I would try to make this point every time I saw them; do not ever lose control of even one dose because it can sometimes take days to get things under control again and it may require taking a lot more morphine to get things back under control. And, it would nearly always cost a night or two of sleep. And the days? Well, they were not pleasant, sometimes barely bearable. For nearly two decades it remained a great contest of reasoning; do I prefer physical pain or stupidity and amplified limitations on nearly anything and everything I tried to do. The limitations were not just physical and mental. I felt emotionally bankrupt much of the time. Empathy, once a strong suit for me was now sometimes easily traded for impatience, frustration, even anger. No I did not need a specific reason to be upset when taking morphine. It messed me up in every way.

Dope makes a person dopey; I didn't like it-

I hated the feelings of stupidity, detachment from reality and the absence of memory. I had memory problems from the beginning but I was enjoying the freedom from the worst of the pain. Over a period of twelve years my morphine doses reached the point that I was taking 45mg of extended release morphine and 7.5mg of immediate release morphine three times a day. I was allowed to take additional doses of 7.5mg immediate release for break-through pain. I tried very hard to not use the extra morphine for break-through pain but sometimes (only a few, it seems) that seemed impossible.

I soon found myself being angry about needing to take morphine but I had no other options that seemed survivable. I hated everything about it except that it helped to reduce my pain level. I fixated on not understanding how anyone could consider taking morphine for anything else but pain. I could not believe that there was a reason that anyone would have for taking it other than to relieve pain. I assumed that everyone would be affected the same as me and I really, really hated to be brain-dead-stupid all the time.

I very much resented having to take drug tests to ensure I was not selling my prescription drugs or giving them away. I made it a bigger deal than it was because I never had anything to hide. I understood the need for the testing and did not express my frustration to any of the people who were helping me. It was not their fault. The thing that always riled me up is the fact that I hated taking morphine because of what it did to me and try as I might (and I did multiple times) I could not understand why anyone would take it for any reason other than to stop pain. I still cannot understand how anyone could possibly see it as a desirable thing to take for any other reason.

I lost me; fears, loss of memory worsens, etc. -
I had tried to stop using morphine multiple times. Each time it was a disaster. Necia finally put her foot down and said that she supported me fully and would help me but only under the direction of a doctor. The pain and drugs as well as the progression of Paget's disease was dictating how I lived my life. That dictated how Necia and (to some extent my family) had to live their lives.

I was losing more memories at an alarming rate. I felt panic most of the time. I met with some of our kids and the grandkids and pleaded with them to be patient with me. I asked them to trust me and to realize that I would never, in my right mind, be cruel to them. I told them that I was losing ground and feared that things may degrade and make me mean. I had witnessed this multiple times in other people.

I asked our kids whose family I could not meet with to please explain my situation to their family as completely as necessary and tell their kids of my fear and ask the kids to remember that in my right mind I would never be cruel to them. I asked all to accept my apology for whatever I may become. It was terrifying to realize that I was (rapidly – it seemed) becoming someone else. I may not have thought much of who I was but I was certainly not fond of who I was becoming. And it seemed that the crazy, stupid, mean stuff just happened. I don't like hiding behind a drug but I admit that while on morphine I just thought, said and did crazy-stupid stuff. Stuff that would leave me feeling unquenchable emotional pain for days as I tried to understand why I had thought, said or did what I did. I am guilty of some really stupid stuff. No, about 99% of the time I would never do any of that stuff if I were in my right mind. But, I had all but forgotten how to think. I was just trying to not hurt and because I had chosen to use morphine to do that I had given up much of my ability to feel, think, responsibly reason. I had traded myself in for a much more defective model.

I made my pleas to the family because I could feel the morphine changing me. My pain was increasing but I told the pain clinic people that I did not want to increase the dose of morphine. I also told the grandkids this because I could feel the Paget's changing me also. Sometimes the tiniest amount of physical effort would leave me feeling sick for a week or more and that also left me feeling quite ornery. I love every one of my grandkids and would never want to hurt them. I had seen people who were living with a lot of pain or who were sick who became very mean, cruel, thoughtless, selfish people. I would try, without letup to make certain that I never became one of those people but sometimes when I was at very high levels of pain I said things that I did not even think about that were sometimes a little edgy. I feared that I was on a slippery slope toward cruelty. As I said, there were times when I did goofy things, said things that I had no idea why I said them. I did hurt some feelings and felt terrible for it. But, I never used morphine as an excuse. I felt that I was still competent and should not hide behind drugs.

This was one of the most difficult things I had ever done. I love my family; my grandkids are all very dear to me and the thought of being cruel to any of them terrified me. I was comfortless about this; I could feel myself slowly slipping away from who I was, who I had always been and I felt I was becoming something I did not want to be. I did not want to die and miss out on seeing them grow up and engage in their adult lives. At the same time I felt certain that I did not want to live long enough to become cruel to them. And as stated above I was already doing and saying hurtful things to others. It terrified me beyond words to feel-hear-see myself careening down this path with adults and face the question as to whether I could do this with others and not have it affect my family similarly. I hated this fact. I hated myself for being such a world-class hypocrite. This drug surely helped me to be miserable. But my physical pain was managed, sort of, and that was something I desperately needed.

Seriously entered distraction mode; it helped -

My life became a very repetitive, predictable boring cycle for weeks at a time. I would take morphine and then go into distraction mode to deal with the pain that the morphine did not fully address. Sometimes the morphine seemed like it was doing nothing to help the pain. At the same time if I was late with a dose I felt the pain start to spike and I would be full of anxiety and panicking until I took the dose and it got into my system.

After several years of seeing the neurologist (my primary care doctor was kept in the loop at all times) he turned my pain treatment over to the local pain clinic which is very good at pain management. Their philosophy was the same as mine: the purpose of pain medication was not to prevent all pain...it was just to make the pain livable. We tried to find a balance between me being crazy because of pain and being crazy because I was so drugged. Mostly we succeeded. There were days when I was crazy in pain but always full of enough morphine to make me stupid. But I realized that I had to have some help from medication or I would be completely crazy...literally.

Side effects -

There are potential drawbacks; side effects, for every medicine. Everyone receives information sheets from the druggist when they pick up their prescriptions. Even if a person buys over the counter medications there will be at least some basic instructions, cautions and list of possible side effects with the medicine.

There is a long list of side effects identified for morphine. One of them is the fact that morphine pretty well shuts down one's colon. Yeah, sometimes it would shut it down for as long as a week. A guy can grow his gut some amount when he is carrying around the last 21 meals. As a kid I used to sort of snicker when I saw advertisements promoting fiber or laxatives. I do not laugh any more. This sleeping colon did not change in nearly 15 years of taking morphine. I was quite sensitive to people telling jokes about "a constipated guy who goes to the doctor and..." Sometimes, even though I did not eat big meals, I got so full I could not feel any hunger for days. This is embarrassing so I will not address this further but it would be errant of me to not acknowledge this while talking about morphine. (I did use several helps for constipation. Some worked sometimes. There were times I thought my colon had died because it was not responsive to various treatments.)

Another common side effect is memory loss. This plagued me from day seven...thereabout, yes, about one week. It made me feel crazy to be visiting with someone and be right in the middle of a sentence and forget what I was saying – sometimes even forget the topic of the discussion (literally). This became worse as time passed and would 'step up' whenever my dose was increased. Friends and family do not appreciate this..."hey morphine guy, we had this same conversation yesterday and you said something different..." "I don't remember." I tried everything anyone suggested to help me with this with no beneficial effect.

This situation was still not satisfactory; being drugged dulled every happy moment in my life -

One of the things I did to distract myself from the pain was think of the grandkids. They are all so bright, and beautiful and so full of life and excited for their future. It was fun to think of their latest communication with Necia and I and always a joy when our children and their spouses would tell us the latest about the little ones and very special when those a little older would communicate with me on their own.

I also found it very satisfying to know what each of our kids were up to and enjoyed hearing about their experiences and achievements. They all make me proud. No exceptions.

Distraction, my main mode of coping -

It is likely that I am "A-D-D"; that worked in my favor because it was natural for me to throw my whole self – every bit of consciousness I had – into recreating special moments of the past. I found it helpful to evaluate certain experiences I had had, sometimes many years earlier, that were not satisfactory and I would try very hard to work through them again and again to see if I could find a solution that would make that experience acceptable if I were to experience it again.

I have always enjoyed music; several genres were more enjoyable than others. If I was really getting hammered with pain loud, discordant music made me very angry. My anger never once helped me to cope or to find any other way to cope or to do mental exercises that were helpful. The opposite was true; whenever I was angry or upset any kind of pain management was impossible. Anger seemed to consume me; demand my full energy and attention and that, so securely, that it was very nearly always impossible for me to create any helpful level of distraction.

Multiple times I would wake up Necia because I was crying in my sleep. She is a beautiful person and always seemed/seems to know how to help me most. Sometimes she would rub my feet or my hands. On occasion she would find a specific 'pressure point' as we have called them, that would actually distract me wonderfully. Sometimes she would find places on my feet or hands that hurt terribly when she rubbed over them. Usually I encouraged her to really get aggressive with those spots. It sounds crazy but sometimes I found that if a different kind of pain were induced that my mind tended to go into overload. It seemed that sometimes that extra pain confused my brain. I still hurt a lot but my mind did not know how to deal with all the pain so I would find myself captivated as I tried to make my mind understand what was happening. That was a wonderful distraction when it worked...sounds stupid to ask for more pain so you will not be as aware of all the pain...or at least not feel the terror that is present when I was sitting between seven point five and ten on the pain scale. This is especially true when the pain was at that level for extended periods of time.

For the first 20+ years following the auto accident my medical care providers always asked me: "How is your pain today; on a scale of 1-10 with 10 being the worst you can imagine." This seemed to overlook how the pain was affecting me, what it was doing to my life so I made the following chart of what it meant when I said a certain number. A few years ago the pain clinic implemented one that was similar; focused on how pain affected a person's life. After all isn't that a big part of the reason pain is a problem? I do not know how to imagine pain worse than I have experienced. I know that a person who has had their arm ripped off in an auto accident must certainly hurt worse than me but I cannot imagine it. So my definitions are defined by my experience.

Pain Levels – My Definitions
Level 1: Pain is noticed but does not interfere with any part of living life.
Level 2: Pain is an annoyance, begins to interfere with thinking as awareness is sometimes there.
Level 3: Pain is constant, I'm always aware of it. Irritating.
Level 4: Pain is interfering with my life. Usually makes me ill to some extent. Keeps me from doing things, even things I like to do. Working around power tools is ill advised.
Level 5: Pain is a pain. I feel spent and at the same time hyped up. Many things are a contradiction. Things I normally like are no longer appealing; food, clothes, organization of a room, movies, television, going for a ride, going for a walk.
Level 6: Focus on the best things in my life and my desires to help them to be comfortable and happy. Death and resurrection and eternal things (family, etc.) give me determination. Anger is often present, not focused on anyone...sometimes it does not focus on the pain as I am always searching for something to distract me. Necia helps me deal with all my pain but by the time things have developed this far her help is essential to me feeling there is an end in sight.
Level 7: After an extended period of time this gets extremely tiresome and I get very irritated; short of patience; feel dark inside and often feel anger toward just about everything. Sometimes (again after an extended time) I start to have feelings like I would like to break things, be destructive. When this goes on too long I still have the troubled desire to do essential things, chores, projects, that are necessary but focusing on anything is a chore in itself. I get little or no satisfaction in doing anything, but I can put a check in the mental box that I did something. Focus on the best things in my life (my family) and my desires to help them to be comfortable and happy. Death and resurrection and eternal things (family, etc.) give me determination.
Level 8: Like with a kidney stone; sleep is difficult to come by. Sometimes tears are present. Depending on how long it lasts it can send me into a "don't care" state where life seems meaningless because I cannot live it. I am severely limited.

Doing simple things can seem impossible. If the stone is too large and is moving fast the pain goes quite high...the same here. It seems that the pain ebbs and flows at this level. I do not know if that is because I am able to focus on other things from time to time and then lose my concentration or what. Focus on the best things in my life and my desires to help them to be comfortable and happy. Death and resurrection and eternal things (family, etc.) give me determination.

Level 9: Sleep is impossible, mind is consumed by the pain; distraction is almost impossible. Usually stomach is so upset it is impossible to take oral medication and keep it down. If it does stay down it usually just sits there as digestive processes stop. Worse than a kidney stone. Cannot sit still; crazy looking for something, anything to take my mind off the pain. I try very hard to see if there are things I can do for those around me to get the focus off my situation. Often tears before the situation is resolved. Focus on the best things in my life and my desires to help them to be comfortable and happy. Death and resurrection and eternal things (family, etc.) give me determination.

Level 10: Sleep is a foreign word that has no meaning. I am not prone to suicide but when the pain is at this level I often think it would be nice if someone shot me or ran over me. This is unbearable; literally makes me crazy. Distraction is completely impossible. At this point utter and complete fatigue must be present in order for the pain medications to bring me relief. It takes enormous quantities of medications to get me sane and in order again. Never without tears. Focus on the best things in my life and my desires to help them to be comfortable and happy. Death and resurrection and eternal things (family, etc.) give me determination.

Examples of distractions -

Here are some of the things I made my mind do to distract me away from being able to only focus on pain. I still rely on these things along with many that are not listed:

- Create poetry. This is much more distracting when I don't write it down until a few hours have passed; then writing it down (typing on a computer) becomes another distraction on its own as I try to deal with my missing memory. This can be done in many ways such as making every line rhyme, making every other line rhyme, make every line rhyme with every second line from it. The possibilities are endless.

- Write stories from my youth in a way my family will enjoy them. Sometimes humorous; sometimes serious. The family seems to enjoy them.

- My memory is a mess but it has provided me many hours of distraction to remember the words to songs or hymns and review them in my mind for hours at a time. Sometimes I try to change the words used in a song or hymn to express my feelings more accurately or completely.
- Composing songs that express my feelings.
- If I am able to get outside I try to find nature at work and to focus on it with intensity. The beauty in nature is a wonderful distraction from pain; watch a bee or a butterfly visit various blossoms and flowers or just flit about. Hummingbirds are wonderful to watch. Some of these distraction activities are enriched by doing a little bit of research about the things I observe in nature. Things like: How many times does a hummingbird beat his wings per minute? How many trips does a bee make to and from the hive during their lifetime? What kind of nest does the bald eagle make and where is the nearest place like that? (I just learned of a place about 15 miles from my home where 20-plus bald eagles winter!) Sometimes the research can just draw me in and away from complete consciousness of the pain for a short period of time.
- It is interesting to look at the rocks in my yard and try to figure out how they got here. I live quite high on a hill and there are many rocks in my yard that have been worn and shaped on a river bottom or at least in a stream bed. Wow! Some of this stuff really gives my mind a place to go.
- When the pickup manufacturers all implemented technologies to make their diesel engines run quietly I spent a bunch of days trying to research stuff and learn about the extra webbing in the engine block, having a single high pressure rail and electronically doing the injection, multiple-stage injection... stuff like that.
- How did the electric motor manufacturers change the motors on shop tools to keep them cool enough when they began to build them totally enclosed? (Making a trip to my tools to see what changed.)
- Trying to think about what people I know are doing and trying to figure out what I can do with my limitations that would make things a little easier for them. When I can do it without just whining about my pain I try to show interest in their struggles. That stuff is a very effective way of gaining new perspectives. To be honest I must admit that I have to be very careful with this or it can generate feelings of guilt.
- It is very uplifting to look at the mountains and imagine trying to hike various trails or go to certain places on the mountains that I can see from my home. I really like looking at the mountains with binoculars.
- It is interesting to look at the limbs people trim off of their trees and count the annular rings and compare the diameters.

- I read a lot of history; mostly war history. I have found it to be a great adventure to try to understand why generals made the decisions they did and see if I can figure out how they could have been more effective. There are many museums that have great libraries on line. The presidential libraries usually have good lectures and enormous collections of oral histories that are very interesting. Much of their stuff is accessible on line – and free.

- My family will do crossword puzzles with me that are a lot of fun and surprisingly distracting. Even if I am hurting enough that my mind is struggling to find distraction and I cannot contribute to the solutions to the puzzles I can enjoy listening to the others discuss and laugh at the humorous things that are learned...sometimes buried in the solutions.

- I have tried to have some contact with each of our children and each member of their families every two weeks. I cannot always do that because some weeks are just so painful that I am not able to be a positive, happy influence in their lives. They are understanding so even if I miss making the contact I am likely to receive an email or text message from some of them.

- Try to remember the name of every kid in my public school experience and try to find a time we spoke and remember what we said. Sometimes I try to remember what their dad did for work.

- I enjoy looking at pieces of wood and visualizing in my mind how they would look turned on a lathe or made into something.

- Sometimes I will count to a predetermined number by threes or sevens or whatever number, then stop at random points and determine what multiple of three, or seven or whatever number it is. So I may begin by counting by threes to 150. When I get to 51 I stop there for a moment until I can say that $3 \times 17 = 51$. If I am extremely tired I have difficulty with this kind of stuff. But if I am lying awake next to Necia and do not want to wake her up I will push through most of the time.

- I am interested in climate and precipitation so I will go to the various Snotel sites the Feds have across the continent and see how various locations are doing for precipitation during that water year. I will extend this to check out the water levels in the huge reservoirs such as Lake Meade, Lake Powell and Flaming Gorge. Most of these sites will have direct links to all of the upstream information such as how many acre feet of water are currently in each of the upstream reservoirs. The Snotel sites all have embedded reporting capability so a person can see the current status against the 30-year average for all measurements. This is very interesting to me and it requires me to do some basic math to calculate a few parameters. If I can get buried in this stuff I find a great distraction from pain. It is interesting to see the electrical power generation at each dam which has generators. It is fun to message the grandkids and tell them that as of a certain time on that day Lake Powell had three trillion gallons of water in it. I get some pretty fun answers in return.

☐ Another great distraction is tracking active volcanoes. There is a site which tracks volcanic activity world-wide in real time. This is a good one for when the pain is over the top because it shows the wonder of this naturally occurring phenomenon. It can distract me with the beauty of the volcanoes while being constantly reminded that these things can be wildly hurtful to mankind. This engages my mind in figuring out how likely it is that a given eruption will reach the domiciles of mankind. There is also an earthquake site that has real-time reporting of "all" earthquakes worldwide. These are never beautiful but the same kind of research is informative and interesting. Sometimes the earthquakes are associated with volcanic activity so the research sort of folds together.

☐ A silly, (maybe) activity for distraction is to take fake trips to/from someplace and see if the various trip calculators agree on miles and time of travel to make the trip. We have family across the country so it is interesting to me to see how soon we could see each of our kids if we left right now. This game has endless possibilities. All one needs to do is add a few in-between points along the way and everything changes.

☐ Sometimes I try to remember the names of people I worked with in industry. I used to think this would be really easy. Things which demand memory are very difficult to do. Sometimes this frustrates me enough that I can not get as distracted as needed. This can actually cause me to anger and make things worse. When I can remember most of them it can be rewarding. Nearly all of my working relationships were good.

☐ I have not been allowed to have a driver license for more than 20 years. I sometimes try to remember places I have driven many times...such as from home to work at the various cities we have lived in. I try to remember, for instance, how I needed to drive to get on the Maine Turnpike and watch all the converging lanes at the on ramps/toll booths. How fast or slow must I travel, when do I brake, etc, etc. This one can last as long as I need it to since there are infinite adjustments one can make. This is not one of my favorites but can help me when I am in a state when the pain is extremely active and I need hours of distraction and use several distractions.

☐ One of the most effective distractions I have is prayer. This can be infinitely variable depending on all of the dynamics active in any given time. This one is not just a distraction but is usually very calming...it may take hours but it will usually calm me. Once calmed I can get very engaged with this and often find myself somewhat disengaged from the pain via distraction. When I am in this mode it is easy to want to pray blessings upon all of my loved ones. If I am going through the lives of each of our twelve grandchildren (and their parents) and I think of what all of our recent communications have been and I can get very involved as I ask the Lord to give them special blessings for their current needs.

- If I am feeling well enough to go for a short walk with Necia and I see an ant pile I will quite likely stop and study it. The behavior of ants is amazing. This was not a pleasant thing to do with the fire ants in Texas. However, I sometimes relive the Saturday I went out to mow our lawn (a couple of acres) and I needed to pull the lawn tractor so it's front wheels were up on the back patio so I could reach under it to change blades. There was a new fire ant hill right where I needed to be (they would appear overnight - literally. I was not feeling very ambitious so I got my little propane torch and lit it and held the flame on the ant hill. I have not been as surprised as this very often but the ants all (ALL) just wildly ran into the flame. Every fire ant in that hill was roasted in less than five minutes and they all volunteered! It amazes me to see a big ant hill and see what the various ants are doing. Check out the large dead insects that one or more of them are carrying down into their hole. Drop a piece of candy, say a Jolly Rancher candy on the pile and watch the ants go for it. Watch how the ants have designated pathways where all the travelers move the same direction. Check out the pathways where they go both directions and usually stay on one side of the path almost like people driving cars on a two way road. Watch the pace at which the ants move and yet they never run into each other. A great distraction if you feel well enough to go outside. Things like this that I can really engage with help distract me a lot.

- It can be distracting to find out about new building materials and learn about those that have great seismic, fire and hurricane ratings...then learn what makes them great. This can be extremely distracting and occupy some time, as much as you want to give it. There are some very amazing things out there.

- One of the fascinating activities I do is, as I read my war history books, it is very interesting to get out my world map and try to find the precise places mentioned in the books with enough accuracy that the geographic barriers referenced in the history are well understood. Challenging!

- When listening to the news I like to pick up on a foreign language word and see if I can tell what it means in English. It is amazing how many words we share and how many more are similar. I sometimes use Google Translate to help me.

☐ It is a very effective distraction to pick up on new words or words I think I know but have never heard used like this, in materials where I have previously seen it. I look up the definitions then create a file on the computer and catalog all the new words and the new meanings for the old words. This is a fun distraction but it can be discouraging because the medicine has destroyed my memory. (Which was never perfect!)

These kinds of things can be changed to whatever interests a person has or would like to have. I have spoken to several other people who are living with great pain and have been told that they also find distraction helpful, at least part of the time, when they are in their greatest pain.

Paget's advances -
I began to feel other effects from Paget's disease. It reached a point that if I did anything that pushed pressure so that it puts pressure inside my head (that) it would set off great pain where the tumors were and where the bones had become thickened. Bending down, and/or picking up a heavy object causes significant pain much of the time. I began to feel sick much of the time. Even moderate activity could have me needing to sleep twelve and sometimes *more* hours at a time. The most ever was 21 hours straight; no drink of water, no going to the bathroom.

Pain is hard on teeth -
Sometimes the pain was reduced to rather moderate levels. It seldom got low enough to not be a huge frustration and problem to my life. Several years earlier, as I have said, doctors had told me that I must leave the work force. I agreed since I was struggling to perform my job at an acceptable level. This was one of the most difficult decisions in my life. I liked to work; I was enjoying my job. I was also very much afraid that I would be fired.

It is true that it has been impossible for me to always distract myself. It is true that it is more difficult when the pain is greater. So sometimes I have found myself just gritting my teeth and trying to hang on. I have broken virtually all of my teeth multiple times by clamping my jaw when I am really consumed with pain. When that level of pain is active I am usually not aware that I do this...until I feel the pieces of tooth on my tongue or bite down such that I push shards down between the roots of the tooth/teeth and my gums. Sometimes I bruise the roots of my teeth and it will hurt to even chew softer foods for a few days.

One of the things I learned along the way is that constant severe pain can cause a person to do things in their sleep that seem impossible. For instance, it seems that people in severe pain could not possibly sleep at all. Extreme levels of pain over extended periods of time can finally wear a person down to the point that they may fall into something resembling sleep. It is not a restful sleep; it is not a peaceful sleep; it is not a sleep devoid of pain i.e. the pain does not go away because a person is so beaten down by the pain, rather the person is just too exhausted to care. So it has been for me over the years of dealing with pain. Not many people have seen me cry from physical pain but I have cried in my sleep from physical pain – multiple (perhaps many) times. I have gritted and ground my teeth in my sleep many, many times with the result of popping off crowns, breaking teeth and crowns, bruising my gums/root tissues for days at a time and doing this repeatedly. My wife has been witness to all of these things while I was "sleeping". I do not know how I stayed "asleep" during these times. One thing that is almost certain is that if a tooth breaks and a shard is driven down along the tooth beneath or above it deep into the root area...that will wake me up.

Morphine lessened this to some extent but I never took enough morphine to allow me to sleep every night or to sleep undisturbed through each night. That much morphine would have made me something like comatose. I did not want that; even with a lot of pain I had reasons to want to be fully conscious. I could still feel and give love. I could still think beautiful thoughts and to a diminishing degree (since morphine robs one of their memory) I could still reflect on beautiful thoughts, beautiful sights, beautiful music, beautiful words...

If a person's intent is to "just forget everything" morphine may help them along their way. I have said and done some things I would give up a lot to forget. However, there remains in my life beautiful people, beautiful sunsets, flowers, birds, butterflies, rocks and natural formations, trees, animals and my family and friends. I guess the short response to this "just forget everything" idea is that the good outweighs the bad. I will try to forget, replace or even overwhelm the bad with a tsunami of good, positive, beautiful things. Why would I want to give up all that is positive in my life to a slave-owner like morphine? Yes, I remain thankful that my wife, my faithful sweetheart, my beautiful best friend and to God our creator that there are natural alternatives to morphine.

Even after 18 months since my last dose of morphine I am still getting "about the same" results in pain relief as I was with morphine: 2-4 days per month when I do not sleep at all because of pain and some episodes of extreme pain that last for hours. However, all the beautiful stuff is still there AND I can enjoy it. I may someday be stung on my nose by a bee that does not want to share the same rose with me as I drink in that wonderful scent and I often (in season) will get showered with lilac flowers as I sniff them and cut off stems to give to my wife. Why would I trade these blessings for a pill that robs me of all of this enjoyment? And why would I trade the views of a beautiful sunset seen through eyes that are wide open and a brain that – even if dealing with pain – is aware of my surroundings...why would I trade that for that dang pill that takes it all from me?

Morphine took away at least some of everything that is good in my life and gave me partial relief from pain. To be sure, I believe that there is a place in our lives, in our society, for opiates but it is not the answer to every stab of pain we feel. And, I am convinced, it is overrated for much of what it is used for. I equate recreational use of opiates to playing tag among the speeding cars on a crowded freeway. A distraction maybe but one with many bad outcomes.

I have no right to condemn others for using morphine; I used it for 15 plus years. Their reasons may be just a legitimate as mine even though different. I do wish that the illegal use could be prevented and that the natural alternatives could/would be embraced by health professionals so that so many people would not suffer from using opiates and no one would die from using/abusing them. The facts are difficult to argue; more than 75,000 people in the US died from opiate overdose between April 2020 and April 2021. I wonder how many are using opiates that have lost much that is good, beautiful, wonderful in their lives because they are using a drug that reduces their pain but costs them so much in return. How many of the overdose deaths were deliberate, people giving up because that pain medication was robbing them of so much that of what made their lives worth living. I'll bet that is a big number.

Endless Pain and thoughts of ...suicide -

One time, it was going on several days when the pain did not let up and it was severe enough that I started to think some dark thoughts. I thought I would try to write something that would be helpful. It happened that my expression was not made pretty by trying to use it as a distraction. As it turned out it was a confession of feeling suicidal.

It was about two o'clock in the morning and I was up and about searching for distraction and accidentally I awakened Necia who immediately got up to see what was going on. I will insert what I wrote about that experience several years ago...

"I reached the point where I felt miserable enough, long enough that life seemed like a great burden. Some people made comments about how nice it would be to be able to not go to work and just goof off like I was sometimes viewed as doing. Only Necia knew of the times that after going out with friends and having a nice time I would come home in unbearable pain. There were a lot of judges. All else being the same (I would never give up Necia and any of our children, even doing a hypothetical what if?) I would have gladly traded them places. Sometimes, if I was having a good day we would go for a little walk or I would get physical with chores in the yard and I would find myself in bed for a few days. This has never gotten better and seems to worsen as the days pass. One fun day working or tinkering in the yard or my shop usually costs me a few days in bed or at least resting."

"One of the things that has been quite frustrating is when the pain got intense enough to make me nauseous. I was extremely blessed when my doctor put me on the kind of "don't puke drug" that disintegrates in my mouth, under my tongue where much of it is absorbed into my body. Often the pain would spike so rapidly that I was puking before the pills I swallowed could do their job and I would just puke them up. That is an amazing medication which I have been very thankful to have."

"For about six months I was sinking lower and lower emotionally. I was far too proud about it and just tried to bury it. Necia did not miss what was happening but I told a few lies and denied that I was in any trouble even though I knew I was a complete mess. Why was it so hard to admit to a mental illness? I was very depressed. I did not abuse others but it seemed that I was sometimes the object of jokes that were no longer funny to me."

"Perhaps everyone has moments when life seems just too big for them. That is where I was. I was becoming consumed with the idea that I had to prepare Necia financially because at the rate my health (how I felt) was declining I figured that my five years were soon to end. I was fighting with myself much of the time. My sweetheart would stop me the minute I started making the 'everybody would be better off if they did not have to baby me frame of mind'. She would tell me that that was not true. She assured me of her love and was very sincere and thorough in her expressions. Sometimes it seemed that she had memorized all the kind things the kids and grandkids had ever said about me (and forgotten any/all of their frustrations with me). She would recite things they had said and elaborate. She was very attentive and very effective."

"Still, I was extremely selfish and would sometimes think stupid, self-destructive thoughts for a while. This kind of thinking made it impossible for me to make any of my attempts at distraction work. This rut was far too deep to climb out of easily. I love my sweetheart and I wish that every person could have a friend like her. She is the master of kindness and unselfishness."

"Sometimes I would get up and walk the house or sit and try to find distraction, so me being up was not overly inconsistent with what I had been doing for years at one level or another. This time I sat there and tried to express myself. It was much easier to do on the computer than in oral speak. Not needing to watch the listener and interpret their expressions and reactions really helped me because being in a lot of pain meant that the pain got most of my attention unless I could develop a sufficient distraction and it drives people nuts to be speaking to me when I am hundreds of miles away."

"I am not a poet but I tried to write it as a poem as part of my attempt to create distraction. I was trying to be honest and speak the truth. This was not a suicide note. It did say that I was getting suicidal but that kind of thinking was stopped when I realized that committing suicide may separate me from Necia for eternity. The last line expresses this."

A Selfish Thought -

When I've made mistakes, done stupid things,
Forgot my lines, or said a word that stings,

When I feel quite worthless, useless too,
Feel full of regrets, mess up all that I do,

When I can't complete the job, or go to work,
When most of the day I think "I'm such a jerk,"

When my head is filled with memories of failing,
When my heart and my mind are flailing,

When I am sharp or thoughtless with someone I love,
When I give in to a bit of pain, ignore God above,

When I take all those pills (now it's rather formal)
And I'm awkward and goofy, can hardly be normal

When I'm whining, complaining and pain is my master,
When I give in to it easier, earlier; faster and faster

When I can't remember things, more than a name or two,
When I don't know what I did or whether I ever knew you

When I fall down for no reason (and pretend I did not),
When I am discouraged, don't want another draught,

When daily I sleep a full half of my life away
When I can sleep much more on any given day,

When I think dark thoughts; what I might do...
I stop it all suddenly; I want to always be with you.

Support and love -

Necia found me standing at the foot of the bed. She immediately got up and came to me, wanting to know what was the matter. I was too emotional to speak so I just asked her to read this "poem" and she would know. She read it then we embraced and stood at the foot of the bed slowly rocking back and forth for a long time. I believe it was as long as two hours. We both wept as we silently rocked back and forth. I did not know what else to do. It felt wonderful to be in her arms. But I felt guilty for, again, preventing her from getting badly needed sleep.

I could not speak. She found her voice first and asked me to wait right there. She said she had bought a gift for me that she was saving for our anniversary which was in just a few days. She left me for a minute and when she returned she had a statue of a couple in a sweet, gentle embrace...the kind a guy needs when he is in pieces and needs someone to hold him together while the pieces healed into their correct places. She had also found a beautiful card that expressed much about our mutual feelings and desires for our marriage relationship. She had framed the card in a way that showed all of the printed sentiment as well as the picture.

She gave these to me as she continued to speak with great love, kindness, acceptance and encouragement. No other person could have possibly been so healing. No one else could have possibly helped me to get out of this rut of self-pity that I was in. I had wallowed out the rut until it was both wide and deep...and as measure by time it was very, very long.

It is a hard thing to climb out of some ruts; the walls are so tall and so steep. It sometimes seems that the walls have a negative slope too, that make the walls of the rut actually lean in toward the center of the rut. For me, on that night, I had to have someone wonderful to steady me as I worked my way up the side of the rut and onto level ground. We spent most of the rest of the night quietly visiting. Eternity could never last long enough for me to forget that night when this beautiful lady loved me back into a desire to give life another chance – loved me back into *really* wanting to live. I pray for everyone who struggles with any hard thing of this type; I pray for them all to have someone who loves them to help them as she helps me. I don't suppose that anyone else would feel *exactly* how I felt because we are all different but I believe that everyone who struggles needs to be healed by love. Love from someone or something such as a pet. For you who are fortunate enough to have a pet to love and to be loved by don't be too hasty to condemn me for referring to pets as 'things'. In my family we often refer to our pets as people. Hearing a phrase such as "Katie (my cat) you surely are an important member of our family" is not uncommon. Neither are lines like this rehearsed. We say them because we feel them. Pets are some of the best examples of giving love – usually unconditionally.

Language of love -

I have been amazed at what beautiful things are said when love is earnestly speaking; quietly and gently comforting; pleading; reassuring; only the sounds of peace. I wish that kind of language for every troubled person. As a troubled person I thank God that Necia was there for me. Everyone needs to know that their life does matter. People who love can always speak with that eloquence and certainty. People who are in great pain, pain of any kind, need to know that their troubles are not greater than their worth. They need to know that that which they need from others is not more than others can give willingly. And the troubled person needs to realize that being belligerent, rude or attacking the person trying to love them will never solve anything, will only multiply the number and size of the problem at hand.

Another lesson I have been learning along the way is that a person who is doing their level best to show their love cannot always say only pretty things; only say exactly what the troubled person wants to hear. Honesty will usually insert itself into the conversation and something that is intended to be kind and helpful can come across as brutal and attacking – if the troubled person is angry or dare I say 'mad'. It is hard to love when someone only wants to fight or hurt the very person(s) who desire to help them.

Speaking as a (working at it) religious person I must forever believe that that night was a gift from Heaven. That experience was the glue that has kept me all in one piece as the challenges have continued to grow.

But...I knew that I must get off of this wretched medicine. I hated it but needed it. I felt that I could not remain sane – if indeed I ever was sane, while I was on large doses of morphine. Also, I could not remain sane if I spent the rest of my life in the intense pain that was then as much a part of me as an arm or a leg. How could I move my life forward? Or should I just coast to the finish line. Some days it seemed like the end could not be too much farther so why not just go through the motions, not knock myself out trying to find and give meaning to my life but just wait for the end and hope it hurries because right now I can barely stand the pain?

As I reflect on this period of time I am nearly overcome with feelings of shame and failure. I didn't really want to die but neither did I know how to continue if my path remained the same. I never made a plan to end my life, never got that serious about "doing it" but the feelings of shame and embarrassment for being such a mess and being such a victim of the pain seemed beyond any measure I could think of. Truly, I felt that even with all of the kindness given to me by Necia; her endless efforts to comfort me mentally, emotionally, spiritually and physically, - even with all of this given so beautifully and consistently, I still could not escape the thought that everyone in my life would be better off if they did not have to make room for me in their thoughts, words or actions – even their prayers.

Self-pity is an ugly thing. Surely it is ugly enough that no one would deliberately choose to lament "woe is me" with each breath, each thought. But I was just about there and I hated it. I hated me all the more because I embraced it even while I hated it. What a liar I had become.

How could anyone who did not have a Necia in their life survive the experience of intense, chronic pain? How could they keep trying at life when as far as one could see was an unending string of days that were full of misery, agony and despair? How could I ever feel useful. How could I ever hold a meaningful place in the lives of all those I loved.

All of this was amplified to an astronomical level by the fact that morphine steals a person's memory/memories. I have joked that I sometimes wondered whose face I was looking at in the mirror while shaving. Yes, that is an exaggeration but prompted by the very real fact that on just about any day I had some very negative failure. I forgot names, places, events, promises, plans. I often groped, unsuccessfully, to recall the events of the previous day. There remain weeks, months, years where it seems special memories are buried in unmarked graves; never to be found; never to be recovered. During 18 months of being clean of morphine only a small number of those unmarked graves have been found.

In the world I grew up in it was not uncommon, when someone was struggling terribly with some horrible foe, for them to be told to "just get over it". I must inform all of those who use this, or a similar line or attitude, to pretend to solve anyone's problem...that is not how life works. That is not how peoples minds and hearts work. And to someone addicted to large doses of morphine that just may be reason enough for them to end it all. Using that line is like kicking the crutches from under the arms of a person with crippled legs and daring them to try to get up. Cruel, brutal, dysfunctional, misguided, completely unhelpful. I agree with you if you are thinking "terribly unkind".

About Pets -

I have long held that pets are wonderful support companions; have mentioned it several times in this booklet. One day it occurred to me that I often felt helped at least as much, if not more, when I was giving them love as when I was enjoying their expressions of love to me.

I mentioned this observation to Necia and she immediately responded in agreement. She said she had read articles that confirmed that to be true. She said that petting an animal releases dopamine and serotonin in significant amounts in the brain of the person petting the animal. She added that she had read that some care centers have even kept cats that roamed the facility freely so that the residents could give/receive love.

Other health-benefits of pets are: lowers blood pressure; lowers cholesterol; improves mood; prevents weight gain by fostering activity; makes one happy; de-stresses a person; protects children against allergies; helps with PTSD... I have read multiple articles which promulgate these claims.

I had no doubt that she was telling me the truth – she always does but since you do not know me you may not believe me so I am including several web addresses where you can verify some of the benefits we obtain as we give love to animals. There are many, many more sites heralding the health benefits of having pets. I hope you will check out some of these sites; I have tried to pick out sites that are likely to endure (stay up) for a long time, here are four:

- ☐ https://www.animalwised.com/benefits-of-petting-a-dog-1529.html (seven major benefits listed)
- ☐ http://conveylive.com/a/Benefits_of_Petting_Animals (nine major benefits listed)
- ☐ https://www.cdc.gov/healthypets/health-benefits/index.html (note that this is on the Centers of Disease Control and Prevention website; multiple benefits listed)
- ☐ https://bestlifeonline.com/pet-health-benefits/?nab=1&utm_referrer=https%3A%2F%2Fduckduckgo.com%2F (this site lists "30 mind-blowing health benefits of pets")

Crying, didn't know it; new things to try -

Life was not easy. I often found myself confused and unable to think coherent thoughts. (More dopey.) This required more and more distraction if I was going to survive the pain. Sometimes while I was just sitting, doing something like watching the birds at the feeder in the backyard, (a wonderfully healing activity) I would become aware that I was crying. (Insert: some of this is redundant but deserves to be said again and again.) How weird! Yes I was in significant pain...even with a belly full of morphine, and yet I was not even aware that I was crying because of physical pain. I would sometimes cry in my sleep. How could I do that? How could a guy hurt that much and not be wide awake and going crazy? How can a guy hurt that much and be awake and not aware that he was sloppy with tears and mucus and crying? How could any of this be true? One answer that I am convinced of is utter fatigue. I proved it again and again; when a person has not slept for days and not rested for weeks their mind/body just shuts down for a while. This old body has ways of demanding time off not just regardless of the pain but also because of the pain. Even admitting this at the time I was taking and hated taking morphine, I remain ashamed that I ever got hooked on it. No I do not know what else I could have or would have done until there were proven natural alternatives.

Throughout these years I often thought of the people who reputedly took opiates recreationally and wondered how they could ever think it was fun, pleasant, or desirable. I wanted to be fresh, alert and able to enjoy things. I wanted to be able to enjoy life and being in a drunken stupor did not allow any of this. Every good thing in my life was cheapened by morphine. It seemed certain that the pain was never going to just go away. Such a miracle did not seem to be in my future.

I must find a way, I thought. But, as usual, Necia was light years ahead of me. As the most loving person that I knew of, she was always doing research on things that will help our family. She had been studying legal, hemp-derived CBD oil; and its properties and benefits for months before I ever even cared enough about it to learn something that may be helpful.

She found one from the hemp plant...neither of us wanted to use the cannabis plant. I only wanted something that would treat pain. I did not want anything that might be mind-bending. I already had that. We never used any CBD oil that was not legal, hemp-derived. (Yes, I realize not all cannabis oil is psychoactive.) And since I first wrote this booklet cannabis oil is now legal in many states – most without a prescription. We made a plan.

Not impressed with first legal, hemp-derived CBD oil -

We agreed that I would take only one capsule at first to check for allergic or negative reaction. I tolerated it just fine so she suggested that we start off at a certain dose which I thought appropriate. I took it for a few weeks. Sometimes it seemed to be taking the edge off of the pain but I never felt it to be a truly effective treatment. It was so iffy and inconsistent that I began to believe that it was just that I wanted so much for it to work that I sometimes talked myself into thinking it was helping. I believed that if it was so occasional in its effectiveness that this was not a real remedy for my needs. So I stopped taking it. And we went back to the drawing board.

Meanwhile I continued to go to the pain clinic. Even when I reported that the pain was really punishing me I would always tell them that I would make the existing doses be sufficient; I did not want the dose increased. They liked that. I always felt support from the pain clinic and my primary care physician. I had taken enough morphine and taken it for long enough that I could have given them a large tome of reasons why I should not have my dosage increased. Each of those reasons would have also been a good reason why I should not be taking any morphine at all. EXCEPT FOR THAT PAIN. Pain is the only reason I could think of for taking morphine and I had to remember that there was one compelling reason for taking it. I am convinced that if there had not been at least one essential reason for me to be taking morphine that I would have not even taken it long enough to get hooked. Without that **one** (I will say the word again) **essential** reason there is nothing worthwhile that came from me taking morphine. Nothing!

A true physician -

One day while I was hurting a significant amount I had a panic attack. I had heard people talk about these and I never wanted to experience one. I did not want anyone I knew to experience such a thing. I am not certain that it was the intense pain that triggered it but *I do know it was not* something that happened by choice. Necia took me to see my doctor who, on one chance in a million, just happened to be immediately available, he very kindly took me into a small room and as Necia stood at my side he took both of my hands in his and softly rubbed them as he gently talked to me. Can a doctor love his patients? I know one that does! He stood there for close to 30 minutes and continued this kind, gentle comforting and assuring treatment. I am quite certain that he could have just given me a shot of something and told Necia to be quick about getting me home before I was so deeply asleep that she could not get me out of the car. I am thankful he did not do that. I did not want to have to rely on yet another drug to keep my feet on the ground. What a person! What an example of human kindness! What a physician!

As the Paget's disease has progressed I have had spells of ataxia. I just fall over. I sometimes do not even know it before I land. One night I fell and struck the back of my head a severe blow. Boy, oh boy did my head hurt! Since the diagnosis of the Paget's tumor in my head and all of the extra bone mass that was present the doctors had told me that it was important that I did not take any blow to the head. The reason? Paget's disease of the bone interferes with the natural and necessary processes of osteoclast and osteoblast, the processes the body has of continuously renewing a person's bones. Paget's causes a thickening of the bones and the new bone material that is put down is thicker yes and denser yes BUT it is also brittle. The very thought of taking a blow to the head terrified me. It was not difficult for me to imagine taking a blow to the head and having a piece of bone driven into my brain. Even with the ongoing thoughts that my life was a messy burden that was foisted upon everyone around me, when it came right down to it I did not want an early exit from life. I wanted to be here with Necia and our family. However, much more frightening to me and much more undesirable to me was the thought of having that imagined piece of bone driven into my brain and leaving me a vegetable. I was impaired enough by morphine; there was no way I wanted to become more helpless. I honestly felt that if such an accident as this did ever occur I definitely wanted death rather than more disability. Especially a disability that demanded more of her.

Since I sometimes pictured myself having been struck a blow to the bones that had the Pagetoid and having the brittle bone break and send shards of bone into my brain, this fall was really traumatic. Necia, our son and I shared the fear that this could happen.

Deceit on steroids -

I was affected enough by the fall that we went to the emergency room. The ER doctor checked on me once (only once and for only about 30 seconds maximum) and was curt and detached and the nurse just kept coming in and telling us that we had to be careful as we got older...blah, blah, blah. We told them that I did not want them to give me any kind of medicine. We told them that several times; even more than that. I have only one other time been treated so disrespectfully. Necia kept asking him to x-ray or CT scan or whatever was most effective - my head to make certain that I had not had a concussion and that my skull had not been fractured. Still the nurse kept up the speech about being careful as we get older and the doctor sat at his desk reading a book or something. If there was another patient in the ER at that time I do not remember them. We could see the doctor from our 'room' and we did not see him get up and go check on anyone.

Necia continued to ask for the x-ray or scan; whichever would do the job best. It seems that this must have gone on for at least two hours. (Afterwards and several times since we have reviewed this experience together and are agreed that it was at least two hours.)

Finally the doctor ordered the x-ray or scan. I do not remember which. When the results came back the nurse said that I did not have a concussion and everything was alright. He essentially said "nothing is wrong, go home and go to bed." Upon release they gave me the standard form that said I should follow up with my primary care doctor within a week.

We saw my primary care doctor and told him that I had fallen and that we had gone to the ER and been told everything was alright. He is a great doctor, very thorough, and he called up the pictures on his computer. He said that not only had I received a concussion but it was a severe one and it would probably take as long as a year to heal. It was important that I take it easy...

Yeah, I could probably take it easy while on a high dose of morphine all of the time. Except that inside I was always in turmoil. For that partial release from severe, and increasing, pain I was watching, feeling, hearing all that was special and wonderful in my life slowly slipping away from me because of the unending stupor that was what my life had become. Sorry, that is not easy. But in the sense of not overexerting myself physically, etc. yes, I could do that most of the time.

After hearing what we told him about our visit to the ER and seeing the pictures he excused himself saying he would return in a few minutes. When he returned he had spoken to the ER doctor who told him that he thought we were just shopping for drugs... What was going on in that man's mind? Do people fake an injury and spend the $100 deductible (just to get into the ER-more for the x-ray and radiologist) and tell the doctor they did not want any kind of drug and that was how they shopped for drugs? And after the x-ray and the radiologist's report (done while we were in the ER) why would he lie and say that everything was okay? Why would he then still tell my primary care doctor that he thought I was on a shopping trip for drugs? Does every person who goes to the ER with an injury get treated this way? Or is this reserved for just those who are taking (legally in my case) opiates? I had a medicine cabinet full of morphine; why would I spend all that money, time and hassle that attends all visits to the emergency room and be treated the way I was in order to get more?

This has been a somewhat traumatic experience. I have wondered if I could ever fully trust a doctor again. (Gratefully I have not found any hesitation in trusting my primary care physician, or the pain clinic.) The issues have to do with other doctors. My situation was that I knew my condition was not improving and it never would improve, this according to every doctor I have ever seen for Paget's disease of the bone – all those who knew anything about it...and to their credit several who went out and studied a little about it between appointments. So, as new symptoms appear or current symptoms become worse can I trust any other doctor? What if a real Paget's disease guru emerges; will I be "able" to go see him/her? Will I ever be "able" to trust him/her? You are correct that out of desperation I may give them a try...perhaps they would be an answer to prayer.

I am thankful we had the follow up with my primary care doctor and that he was thorough. I was beginning to know how other people felt when doctors accused them of trying to get drugs by acting some part. Grrrrr! Maybe some doctors will suspect bad motive on your part. It is certain that not all will.

I include this story in this booklet to be honest with the reader. Doctors are not all the same. A person may need to go to more than one doctor to get the help they need. I was very fortunate to have a very caring and capable primary care doctor. I always felt he had my best interest in mind in all he said and did. Please don't give up if you are taking opiates and have to try several doctors to find one who truly cares and is entirely competent who will help you get off of the sinking boat of opiate use. One of my sons is an MD. I spoke to him about this at some length and he reminded me that all doctors are people too and they they also have bad days and that sometimes they are accused, abused and otherwise treated contemptuously. That prevented me from suing IHC and probably ruining that man's life. On one or two extremely difficult days I have almost reconsidered my decision. The several people who know this story, some quite knowledgeable in law, have nearly all told me that it would be an easy win in court.

More bad thoughts -

This letter to my sweetheart was written some days after the night she found me standing at the foot of the bed wallowing in self-destructive thoughts.

Dear Pretty Lady,

It has only been a few days since I shared my fit of agony with you. That time with you was beyond anything my command of words can describe. Truly, I had never anticipated such a moment in my life, even though my life is the perfect storm for incubating the things which made it rain. That is what happened, I rained tears. You have always known that my emotions ride near the surface and manifest themselves at the most inconvenient of times. I have always appreciated the fact that you have allowed my emotions to overcome me and not even once made me feel badly or embarrassed when I did rain.

Back to the night referenced. Having watched a few people lose their connection to reality and with it the understanding of what transpires in their lives. It has made my heart ache for them and for their caregivers. Of all the questions I have that remain unanswered and that trouble me it is why people are given such hurt as attends these circumstances. It breaks my heart to even think of this. The only people I know of that are in this situation are very good people. I cannot bring myself to believe, for even the shortest of moments, that these things happen as a sort of judgment for how they live their lives; both the victim of the illness and their families and caregivers. Seeing these things happen to very good people, watching their world quietly slip away from their conscious, comprehending state and knowing my profound inadequacy at living a life which would make me deserving of anything remotely as good or positive as them...if goodness is a factor, I feel somewhat helpless and absolutely terrified.

As I expressed to you the extreme and complete terror filling my heart and mind as I consider what may happen to me, I shudder. My fear is founded on what happens to me or what may happen to me, myself. It is very selfish in that way but it goes far beyond that. I do not want others to be consigned to care for me in such a state. That too is selfish. I do not want for you to tell me that you love me and me not be able to understand all that that means. I do not want for there to ever be even the most remote chance that I will ever speak to you words of unkindness or hurt; I have seen it happen. Even the thought of these things happening just consumes me inside as if my insides were on fire. It makes my head feel like it is caving in from some external weight greater than I can carry.

These thoughts come to me in intervals short and heavy with fear and as I said terror. On the night mentioned I was in a state of dissolution. My mind was riveted on these thoughts and potential state. As terribly tired of taking large doses of morphine as I am...and the consequences of what happens every time I try reducing the dose, I feel like I am in a prison that has no door, no key, no secret way in or out. It is in the truest sense a prison.

Being very aware of how this medicine affects me and the effects on my mind terrifies me. With the situation now being that, (at least at that time) some doctors will not even consider me even reducing my dose I am completely helpless to escape the problems that morphine, along with all the other drugs, cause in my life.

And yet taking those drugs, knowing their affect on me gives me hope. Perhaps my fears are unfounded and I will not ever be required to join that group of nice people, good people who have their light flicker and then go out before their bodies give up. But since the extent of the memory loss and the frustrating and completely terrifying thing it is that some days I cannot, even hold a thought or maintain a conversation which I am very interested in, I am always left wondering if my die is cast and I am following others into that dark prison. On my best days, escaping from that captivity pummels me and consumes me. I do not want to lose the ability to recognize you, our children, our grandchildren or to not be able to exchange greetings and expressions of love. I do not want to lose the ability to reminisce about special memories. I do not want to ever forget even one thought of you and the deep love we share. I am resentful of the way the drugs alter my usually calm and kind nature and add becoming an unkind person to possible...if not likely consequences. I have already spouted off against others several times for which I am immediately sorry. But words are like sharp daggers and usually pierce the hearts and minds of those who receive them. Even when the daggers are removed, unless the parties involved are mature and are able to completely forgive they leave scars.

This has become a very long expression of thanks to you for your expressions of love on that miserable...then beautiful night. As my emotions overfilled my heart and you held me in your arms and assured me that things are alright as long as we have each other. For what must have been two hours you kept gently, lovingly assuring me that that is true; everything will be alright as long as we have each other. (That has always been said between us; I needed my certainty to override my terror.) You answered each of my concerns, all of them with that same assurance. Even as you held me all my fears percolated to the top and each evaporated as they were confronted with your beautiful, kind assurances. What power you have! What power your heart has! What power your words have! As I told you multiple times that night I am utterly and completely terrified of what the future may bring into my life, into our lives. But I do believe that as long as we have each other everything will be alright.

As long as we have each other everything will be alright and that is true because we love each other. And I do love you; how I truly love you.

-Yours forever, Hubby

How blessed I am to have this angel as my constant companion. What about all the other people who are hurting? What about those who are treating their hurts, their pain with opiates – prescribed or otherwise? Who is helping them? How are they dealing with their pain...yeah, all the pain caused by messing one's mind up with opiates? Certainly I cannot possibly be the only person on this planet who got messed up by taking morphine (or other opiates). I felt desperate to escape the clutches of this drug. Do they?

The world's worst wake up call -

Sometimes I would stand in front of a mirror and feel the places on my head that were beginning to increase a little bit in size and were beginning to show signs of slightly reshaping my skull. It is important that a person know that our brains do not feel pain. Surgeons can open up our skulls and if proper deadening (what a word) is in place to prevent the pain sensation in the skin, muscles and bone they can do brain surgery without using any more drugs. I have been told this by multiple doctors. I have never thought that my brain was hurting because of Paget's disease but I feel like an expert at feeling bone pain. I have also learned how to whine more than a little bit. But I got a terrible wake-up call at one point in time when I was feeling sorry for myself. I did not pray with the demand to know "why me!" No, I have never asked that question because I figured that if the Lord decided that I needed to learn something by this, his purposes may be important for me to understand but I have not felt that I necessarily deserved better than the next person.

Back up to that wake-up call. I got a wake-up call of the worst sort. While I was focused on learning how to manage my own pain, my beautiful sweetheart, my best friend, my everything was diagnosed with cancer. The doctors said it was "a very aggressive kind" and would require some very potent chemicals doctors used to make up their cocktails for her. She was on this treatment for a full year. This nearly broke me. My prayers for her often ended up with me pleading for the Lord to spare her and allow me to take on that burden for her. Those prayers were met with what seemed a resounding 'NO'. She did not know of my request for the cancer to leave her and afflict me. Years later I learned that she was asking God to remove my pains and problems and give them to her. What an amazing person. Other than my faith in God my choice for her to be my life-and-beyond-companion was my greatest help, my greatest strength.

I was struck with how she must be feeling; spending her life-force to look after me and having the table turned so that she was facing this struggle without any of my problems being lessened. During the wee hours of that night I wrote her this note. Writing it was one of the most powerful medicines I have ever taken. I felt the full gamut of thoughts during the several hours that it took me to compose this letter. When completed, it would fill me with a determination to get outside myself and try my best to serve her with a commitment equal to her selfless caring for me.

Again, I do not fancy myself as some great writer. I do know that I am usually much more able to express myself effectively when I write than I am when I am just running off at the mouth. So, I sometimes write when important things need to be said – especially to her.

Here is what I wrote to her the day (night) she was diagnosed with cancer...

Dear Pretty Lady,
Today -

For 40 years I have marveled at your beauty. You won me completely. Although the reasons were many your beauty, your good looks, have never been lost to me. Yes, you were all a fellow could ask for; more than most could even imagine. Indeed there were suitors in-waiting, waiting to see if we would ever part.

During the ensuing years the experiences of life continued to reveal hidden beauties; characteristics and traits of personality and character that only made you more beautiful. Along with the experiences that were desirable, wonderful to be part of, there were also those more revealing of character and courage.

Bringing children from heaven to earth cost you your youth. Still, it made you more beautiful; ever so much more desirable. The beauty and wonder of each newborn child inspiring a sense of awe and an anxious silent plea that we could raise him/her such that the Lord would bring us back to His presence as a family. We became ever so much closer as the bonds of love that arrived with each child tangled themselves in enduring knots around our hearts. There was no escape. Nor has there been any desire to escape.

So today as you sit beside me I am once again reminded that you are so much more than I could have ever imagined any person could be. You are everything that attracted me to you. You are everything we have learned over the years. You are everything we have experienced during those years. You are everything we have dreamed over the years. You are my past. You are my future. You are my happiness. Truly, you are my everything.

Today we learned that soon a doctor, in an attempt to preserve your life, will remove some part of your body. Oh how I have desired that you would never have this experience. How I have prayed that God would work his mighty miracle and heal you by His power alone. How my heart aches as I see you continuing to push forward insisting on caring for others with barely an acknowledgment of your own needs. Yes, through it all you remain the same; unselfish, intelligent, kind, determined. You remain my everything. The doctor will not, could not, remove anything that will make you anything less than my complete everything. Today and tomorrow.

I love you with all my heart,
- Hubby

Answering the call; better distractions -

As I said, her experience with the treatments for her cancer was severe because the cancer was so aggressive. I honestly believe I could never have survived that treatment. But she was strong, positive and always focused outwardly. I was often ashamed that my pain so often, and so much, turned me inward. Oh yes, I was making progress in my collection of ways that helped me to endure the pain but I also became aware of just how dangerous it could be if I lost control of my concentration on distractions and allowed my focus, my intense focus, to drift out of control and gather thoughts about the pain. It was disastrous when that happened. All that focused attention landing with a negative force that could bring me to my knees.

Landing on my knees was a good thing. It put me in the perfect posture to do the only thing that was sufficiently strong to burst the horrible bubble of self-destructive thoughts that would inevitably accompany a fit of self pity which was now mixed with increased guilt. Some of my acquaintances do not believe in God for the very reason that so many of his children have suffered so much and, to them it seems He has abandoned them...if He was there in the first place... I reflected on this often; I am certain He is there and that He is watching over us. In my most desperate moments my visits with Him were what could call me away from selfish and destructive thoughts. I have no doubts that there is purpose in whatever we suffer. We also have some personal responsibility to learn from our experiences. This is a rather frustrating truth when we are so completely overwhelmed and we cannot just put on a Band-Aid or spray a little pain relieving stuff on a small wound and be completely okay. No, that will never do and blaming Him for stuff is never helpful.

A somber, grateful reflection on history -
Many times as I have struggled with my pain and been at the point of wondering if I could ever win this battle I have found comfort in the terrible/beautiful story of our Lord's suffering for all of us. I have wondered that I could sometimes struggle to find purpose in my own, small measure of suffering...certainly very small, almost non-existent pain compared to his and yet so enormous and difficult for me. Knowing about his love and many times feeling it has changed me.

Otherwise it seems that all was just a waste; the pain, suffering and many times the feeling of being so very alone at night when I was the only one awake in the house and teetering on a breaking point. Yet, now thankful that He has never abandoned me.

Eternity yawned wide sometimes, ready to swallow me up in a darkness devoid of purpose and meaning. Then as the hymn declares, "The Morning Breaks, The Shadows Flee..." Prayers are answered and sufficient strength is infused into my soul as I once again acknowledge that even though I do not always understand or even remember why things are as they are, there is a worthwhile purpose. I will survive this day and do my best to not murmur. And I will do my best again tomorrow.

I believe this is why AA and others declare that one must have a belief in a Supreme Being/Power to have success in their program of overcoming addiction. Certainly I could not manufacture the relief, the liberation, the power, the healing, the love...His love and the living, loving devotion of my sweetheart. Never, in ten lifetimes could I have traveled this path alone and won.

Essential support -

With all that said there is much to learn. Following the night in which I was feeling suicidal my beautiful wife joined hands with Heavenly Father and began a healing sequence of words and action. I wish every person had a friend and companion such as she is. I have been witness to pure love – I have been the recipient of pure love; His and hers. To have such a companion is a blessing beyond measure.

I fear that my frequent references to her goodness, kindness, helpfulness could really be discouraging if someone reads this and they do not have such a companion, friend...etc. Please forgive me for that. She and I have discussed this multiple times and agreed that there are other ways; to find that love. Special friends, pets, volunteers in addiction recovery programs and even some professionals. The old statement that 'a dog is man's best friend' is based on someone's experience and is endorsed by the experiences of untold numbers of others. I have watched many others' experiences (and my own) with pets and that assures me that there are pets which provide love and support to their owners (I want to say "best friend"). I currently have a cat which has been a friend to me and my family for the past 18 years. In our household of three adults she is the object of our affections much of the time.

It is not just the love pets give to us that is therapeutic. They also lift us and heal us and help us as they allow us to make them the object of our affections. Animals are so appreciative of any love we give to them. We can learn to love them such that we can forget some of our pain as we focus on their comfort. Giving love to them helps us to shrug off some of our own pain. Some will attest that our pets are better friends than other humans because our pets are more dependable, more unconditional in giving love and they return love in multiples of what they are given. I hope you have looked at the web sites I provided earlier on the benefits pets can provide to us. I hope if you have or get a pet that you treat them kindly. They will almost assuredly return your love in multiples...unless your pet is a snake. I am terrified of snakes and don't believe they can give love...nor spiders...I am distracted – can you tell?

Time for an oil change -

Not to be beaten, Necia had been out researching for weeks, perhaps three or four months. She found a different brand of legal, hemp-derived CBD oil that also had extracts from two plants which were known for their use in treating pain and anxiety. (no THC)

She is exceptionally observant and she was well aware of my anxiety when in a lot of pain. She also found a homeopathic formula that is simply labeled as "Anxiety Relief".

She started to give me the new kind of legal, hemp-derived CBD oil with the anxiety relief formula and three different essential oils. Wow! The effect was wonderful. The pain did not all go away and sometimes it seemed like I was still standing in an ocean of pain. But it was a great help; <u>I believe, for me, as effective as the morphine</u>.

One day, following a week or two of serious thought, very serious, I announced to Necia that I must get off of morphine very soon. She, as the wise one among us, responded that that was a thing which she would support me in doing as long as I was being able to deal with the pain without it destroying me. She asked me to make certain that I was not attempting to do something that would tear me apart. She also insisted that I do it under a doctors supervision. She was right about this. I tried to go off of another medication cold turkey and it put me in such panic attacks that even after I went back on it I spent a year sleeping in a recliner because every time I laid down flat in bed I would go into severe panic attacks. Weird but true!

Making a schedule -

I had thought a great deal about this; I was certain that I must do it. We discussed how we should proceed. I had told the guys at the pain clinic that I wanted to get off of morphine and asked them for some guidelines about choosing how to do it. Using their input we agreed on this schedule:

1. Take 15mg out of the dose that was my first daytime dose for one week.
2. Take 15mg out of the dose that followed noonday for one week.
3. Take 15mg out of the bedtime dose for one week.
4. Iterate on steps one through four.
5. Iterate again on steps one through four.
6. Take 7.5mg of immediate release out out of the morning dose.
7. Take 7.5mg of immediate release out of the afternoon dose.
8. Take 7.5mg of immediate release out of the bedtime dose.
9. If necessary quarter the 7.5mg of immediate release tablets and take them at four hour intervals then eliminate them one at a time.
10. Celebrate that I am no longer a prisoner to morphine.
11. Talk with the guys at the pain clinic about XXXX. A medication which I had learned about during the process of getting off of morphine. (To this day this has turned out to be unnecessary.)
12. Make certain that I never knowingly take morphine again.

D Ts (delirium tremors)-

Multiple times I had to stay on a dose for two weeks before stepping down again. As I have mentioned before, once, a long time ago I had traveled somewhere hours away and forgotten to take my emergency doses which I carried in a medical container in my pocket. I found it shocking that I could feel the way I did just because I did not take a few pills - tiny pills. I would never again find even a modicum of humor when a movie scene portrayed some poor soul having delirium tremors. I do not require any explaining to understand exactly how they feel.

I have seen how Hollywood depicts the D Ts, usually trying to make it humorous. There is nothing funny about feeling like your skin is trying to shed itself; almost an itch but nothing that any kind of rubbing, scratching...no matter how hard or vigorous can even begin to affect. There is nothing funny about sweating like you are sitting in a sauna with a runaway heat control. There is nothing funny about your nose running like a hose. There is nothing funny about the only thought in your mind being on relief from this torture from getting your pill or being hit by a train. There is no compromise – just stop this horrible experience; whatever you have to do.

Pain management continues to be essential -
I was dosing every eight hours and I missed a dose. About five or six hours later I was in trouble. First my skin started to crawl. By the time I was 12 hours since taking a dose I was, literally, going nuts. Truly I was out of my mind looking for something to save me from being consumed. It got worse and worse as the time passed. My nose was running 'like a garden hose'. I was sweating profusely. I was panicking and quite literally dancing around. I could not force myself to be still. I could not stop. Had my life depended on it I could not have stopped.

On the way home I could not sit still. Having the seat belt even just lying lightly across my shoulder had me wound so tightly that I nearly snapped. I must have taken nearly enough steps to walk home as I moved my feet constantly, irritatingly across the floor mats of the car. I believe a person could go insane dancing the DT dance. I am certain of it.

The last time I saw a neurologist he said that the Paget's had surrounded my entire inner skull. To me it looked like a white band about a half-inch thick. The thicker bone with the tumor was still very visible and if possible my brain had moved a tiny bit farther to the left side of my head. That seemed strange because by that time I also had at least one Pagetoid on the left side of my head.

The time had arrived for the first reduction in dose; it went sideways. I dropped the first 15mg from the first daily dose. I went a day or two before I started to consciously and constantly be aware of the heightened pain. Still I bragged around to my kids that I was running on less morphine. I was really pleased with myself.

About a week had passed since I had been taking a lower dose for one dose each day. Then I was bragging to someone again. Necia pulled me aside that night and very apologetically explained that after multiple days at the lower dose she had resumed giving me the prescribed dose. She said that it was breaking her heart to watch me during the day as I dealt with the awareness of the greater level of pain. She also said that I was crying in my sleep and that made her hurt terribly.

Our pain affects others -

No, I did not get angry, not even frustrated; but it did discourage me a little bit. If a 15mg lower dose on one dose per day affected me as it did, how could I possibly get off of morphine? She then told me that she would support me in whatever I truly wanted to do but I needed to be aware of what I was doing, how I was acting day and night. She was not complaining about how I was acting; she was wanting me to understand what I was doing so she could help me and so we could change things if necessary. We agreed on full disclosure – both directions. No secrets. I am a blessed person to be her husband. I didn't even know I was crying in my sleep. (Maybe that is because I was asleep – seriously, I did not know that a person could cry from pain in their sleep, tears and all, and not have them wake up.)

As I considered this I recalled numerous times when I was crying from pain when I was awake and was not aware of doing so until I felt the tears running down my cheeks. Sometimes the pain was so great that it seemed to put all of my thinking on hold. I could not even think enough to remember that we had found things that could help the pain. I could not even think enough to remember to tell Necia that I needed help. Usually she would see from my behavior that I was in trouble and would ask me enough questions to verify the nature of the problem and either get for me or tell me where stuff was and what I needed to take to deescalate the crisis I was in.

Summary of withdrawal problems (symptoms) -

There are numerous symptoms one may experience during withdrawal. Most of them hit me pretty hard and lasted through most of my withdrawal period of five and a half months. This is not fun stuff. Following are two lists of many of these symptoms; one for those symptoms that show up in as little as 24 hours followed by a list of symptoms that show up beginning a day or two later. I indicated how these symptoms affected me in terms of intensity. I cannot describe the misery that came with nearly every one. Honestly, most of these symptoms would hit me with enough strength to knock me off my center. Meaning they affected me enough to really interfere with me doing anything which required my mind to be clear. While I was reducing dose size I was usually struggling to participate 'normally' with just about everything and everyone.

Withdrawal symptoms that began early on (usually beginning in the first 24 hours).

- ☐ <u>Eyes tearing up.</u> This is extremely odd to yawn, and yawn just because one's body says to yawn and the only obvious or observable affect is to have tears running down one's cheeks. This tearing up is massive and did not require a yawn but the yawns really amplified the tears; it is the kind of tearing up some would desire when they get some dust in their eyes. It often seemed enough to float a small boat. This is different than the tears from crying because of pain. I was once subjected to tear gas as a joke from a friend. The tears from withdrawal were every bit a real and voluminous as they were from the tear gas. And they were just as impossible to stop on command.

- ☐ <u>Muscle aches.</u> The worst of the muscle aches were in my upper arms. It was worse than any muscle pain I have otherwise experienced in my life. This did begin immediately and lasted for the first four and one half months of my escape. Sometimes my arms hurt so badly that it required focused, deliberate direction from my mind to be able to even lift my hands from my waist to any height above my naval. This was almost constant and amazed me that when I started ramping down my doses of a pain medication that I could hurt so much. Massaging and applying heat made little difference, if any. This is one side effect from withdrawing that I feel lingers. From time to time this visits me again and is just as real. There is no warning that tomorrow will be such a day and nothing today that says that yesterday was such a day. It just happens.

- ☐ <u>Restlessness</u> appears as an unlikely-sounding symptom. However this interfered with my sleep the majority of the time all the way through mid-June; four and a half months into my journey. I believe this restlessness is closely coupled to the endless anxiety.

- ☐ <u>Anxiety</u> was present most days throughout the first four and a half months. Sometimes it diminished for a few hours immediately after dosing but would come back within two or three hours. This was treated with the homeopathic "Anxiety Relief" tablets which brought relief and sometimes freedom from this problem for some hours. This is a terrible feeling that tries to defy distraction so any help has been something to be very grateful for. It took me tremendous concentration to deal with this using distraction. Having something physical to do, even something like household chores was often a good outlet for this. It did not just wipe the anxiety away but it allowed some outlet while being distracted by the thought process accompanying, or directing oneself in the physical activity.

- ☐ <u>Runny nose</u> is another bodily function that is hijacked by the withdrawal process. I experienced much of this. Even in the final two weeks of withdrawal my nose would just start dripping. Both nostrils. I describe this elsewhere.

- ☐ <u>Sweating</u> is yet another bodily function that withdrawal hypes up to unexplained levels. I was often soaking wet with sweat sitting in my summer pajamas in a room that was 70 degrees F. This did not ease off until I was within the final two weeks when I was only taking 3.75mg/four hours, going to zero mg.

- ☐ <u>Sleeplessness</u>. About half of the time when I took a step down in dose I would lie awake at night even when I was completely exhausted. This occurred even when I was not feeling troubled or worrying about other things. It is brutal to be so wiped out and not be able to sleep. This happened consistently through my withdrawal journey. I had read about sleep deprivation used in prisoner of war camps as a means of torture or as a means of trying to break prisoners. It would work!

Withdrawal symptoms that occur later, symptoms which can be more intense, begin after the first day or so. They include:

- ☐ <u>Diarrhea</u> came in waves. This is a strange symptom since I had spent 15 years being severely constipated by the morphine. Maybe once or twice a year during those years I would be 'moved' by illness or in response to something new in my diet. I welcomed this but not ongoing. It was sometimes ongoing during withdrawal but several of the episodes were beyond any experience in my life. One episode lasted for three days and during that time it felt that my colon was tying itself into a very tight knot so that even when my body was literally expelling explosively I felt like my body was unable to clean itself out. It was as if my body was passing my colon...not just the contents but the colon itself. Terribly distressing and nothing helped except the passage of time and the involuntary spasms which would end only after some hours passed. One time it took an entire day at this brutal task. Some doctors say that a person on morphine for an extended amount of time may have retention of as much as 30 pounds of fecal matter in their body. I believe this could be possible.

- ☐ <u>Abdominal cramping</u>. I had only a limited amount of this beyond what seemed to just be a part of the diarrhea.

- ☐ Some people get <u>goose bumps</u> on their skin during withdrawal. I did not.

- ☐ <u>Nausea and vomiting</u> were very much a part of my withdrawal. Just as they have been part of my pain. Your doctor can prescribe a medicine that will dissolve under your tongue in about 30 seconds that (in my case) stopped these monsters in their tracks. As quickly as the nausea came and the viciousness with which it struck would have had me kneeling at the toilet for hours without this medicine. I would sometimes think that for certain I was coming down with the plague or some other terrible disease because of the nausea. I believe that my nausea moved to actually puking only a few times whenever I was able to use this medication. I already had a prescription for this medicine to use with my migraine issues. It is truly a Godsend. I always kept several of these tablets (in their foil packages) under my pillow; at my computer; where I sat to eat; where I sat to read; and where I watched television as well as several in the aluminum medicine container in my pocket. Being away from this medicine always put me at risk of having a nausea/puke attack. I have significantly reduced my use of this medication but still count it a blessing to have.

☐ <u>High blood pressure</u> did become a factor in my case. My insurance company made a digital blood pressure kit available to me so I could track my blood pressure. After I had dropped my doses by 15mg my blood pressure raised by about 15 on both diastolic and systolic measures. This continued at this level for about three months. I was delighted to know that my increase in blood pressure was temporary but I still have a bit of work to do to completely beat this thing down because of the status of my health generally. Now after being clean for 18 months my blood pressure is just about normal for a healthy person of 69.

☐ I did not note my <u>heartbeat ever being rapid</u> but many, perhaps most, people do.

☐ I did not ever check the <u>dilation of my pupils</u> but it is a common symptom of morphine withdrawal.

☐ <u>My vision became blurred</u>, at times, and I found that I required my reading glasses virtually all of the time in order to see well enough to read anything that is smaller than number 12 font. Sometimes I could not even clear my vision to read 12 font. That got better as I neared the end of my journey.

Yuh Gotta Wanna -

If my experience means anything, it will be impossible for someone who does not truly and honestly want to get off of an addiction to ever do so. This is very hard and torturous work and a person will experience things not common to a peaceful life. I am not certain I can describe the D Ts in a way that is understandable to anyone who has not had them.

Unless a person really wants to get off morphine the D Ts will break them...they nearly broke me several times and I truly wanted to be off of morphine. What we see in movies is a modest example of the real thing. A person must feel a frustration, perhaps an anger or maybe it is a sense of loss of their life that makes them resent the drug. Otherwise I believe they will not re-engage in getting off of morphine after a bout or two with the D Ts.

If a person has these intense anti-opiate feelings, I believe, they will come back of their own will and try again, and again, and again. They will take the lead and tell their support person, pet, group... whomever, that they are ready to try again.

Try again –

Several weeks or months later (after I had tried and failed several times and felt I had taken a huge step backwards) I told Necia that I really had to get off of morphine before it killed me. I was certain it would. Even if it did not put me in the proverbial 'pine box' it was progressively killing my desires for life; for association with others; and for wanting to be something good. I was at the point that much of the time my highest priority in life was simply to not hurt. It was all about me. That remains a very big deal to me. I detest this feeling. Working hard to get rid of it.

We agreed that the original schedule we had made was the correct one to follow. It reflected the advice or description the pain clinic gave us. Stand by for a bit of a circus...

I think it is instructive that Necia left me in charge – promising that she would provide my medications in the doses I wanted as long as it did not violate the doctor's advice. Since we did this at home my prescriptions had never changed. She has, from time to time, queried me about the pain as she has seen me struggle, but she never nagged or badgered me to stop the pursuit of my goal; nor did she resent the goal itself even though it demanded much of her. Don't misread this; she very much wanted to be involved. She was not trying to be in charge or to be controlling. However sometimes she did have to be the referee and call a foul. She kept strict track of my dosing times; when cutting doses 15 or 20 minutes can have an astronomical effect. Her keeping track of and ensuring the accuracy of doses was an essential help to my success.

The first dose adjustment went well. I felt the increased pain but the fact that I had made it was a really big deal to me. I had only taken two weeks with one dose and one week each with the other two daily doses which meant that it took only four weeks to reduce 15mg on all of the daily doses of morphine week. This was a success worthy of celebration. It was extremely difficult. To accurately describe it would be a repetition of D Ts, all of the major effects of quitting an opiate addiction and numerous mental traumas as I tried to master distractions. Yes I said distractionS.. That capital S became a huge factor. I was now learning and using distractions for pain and for the withdrawal symptoms.

Sometimes I was trying to distract myself from pain and withdrawal at the same time. I know Necia would have kept her word and would have allowed me to increase my dose...go back to the level I had just come down from. That comforted me but she was one of the reasons I wanted/needed to get off of morphine. I wanted her all back. She had never abandoned me or withdrawn from me but morphine did not want me to have her. Morphine is the stereotypical "woman scorned". Morphine wanted all of my attention and all of the cursed pain was on her side. Morphine whispered in my ear things like "just take another 15mg and you will feel better. You did it before and it worked for a while; go ahead, you know it will still work, especially since you are coming from a lower dose". How I hated that; knowing I could easily escape more of the pain for a while at least, some of the withdrawal symptoms and I had to say no to be true to my true self. I had to be true to the part of me that loved my sweetheart, my Necia, and our family.

This is not easy -

During this time there were several significant events. One night the pain was especially severe and it caused me to cry. She and one of our sons and I sat and visited while I cried for an hour; probably a couple of hours. I was grateful for their companionship and appreciated that she asked me exactly one time if I needed to take an additional half of my immediate release morphine for breakthrough pain. When I responded with a "no thanks" she took my hand and rubbed it firmly but gently and began to help me to find distraction. Neither Necia or our son even commented about my crying beyond that. It was always complete acceptance and support for me to reclaim my freedom; to find myself again. I don't know if they knew I was actually reclaiming them again. I was, with their help, chasing off that old hag, morphine so that I could fully claim them. I wanted my family to have claim on me rather than me claiming morphine.

This is gross but may provide some worthwhile insight: during this cry-fest I did not use a box of Kleenex or a roll of toilet tissue; I used a roll of paper towels. The tears and the running nose both required lots of drying power!

More about being reasonable, not rushing it –

On several other occasions I pressed the agreed schedule a bit aggressively and found myself in withdrawals. Talk about anxiety, fear, desperation, panic, much more panic! I wondered how many people had been destroyed by withdrawals. If the D Ts were severe Necia would give me (or at least offer me) a half-tablet or 7.5mg of immediate release morphine and talk with me, rub my hands and or my feet. She never tried to change my mind about getting free of morphine. She only asked what she could do to help me. A time or two, maybe three, I may have been in a state to do violence (not hurt Necia or our son – more likely just break something) in order to express my need to get more morphine. That was my physical response but my mental resolve took the day. I was truly an addict. Again, all of their help was kind, positive and was truly supportive of my long-term goal. I had full realization that people who work with those who are trying to overcome addiction must all be loving, kind people. I am also certain that those who do this work must also be persons with strong resolve in order to be effective. There are not many times I have felt lower than I would feel when I was being controlled by addiction. I could not watch people struggling like that day after day. Knowing how they were feeling would bring out the decision from hell: do I give them their drugs so they can escape this suffering or do I help them to hang on to their determination to quit their addiction so they can have their life back? One is immediate "pleasure", the other is delayed, but lifelong, pleasure.

I do not profess to understand how morphine works but it amazed me that I could be so completely controlled by those pills. I have never had withdrawals when I went too long without ice cream!

It was as predictable as gravity; I had withdrawals with each reduction in dose. Most of the time it would take me two or three days to calm down and to go to sleep soundly. I would go to bed as usual and mostly just lie there waiting for sleep to find me; I could not find it. Some times it did not find me for 36 hours or more. Necia would tell me every time that for at least the first two days following a reduced dose that I would run around in the bed all night. There would be more pain – sometimes quite a bit more. Always I have wondered why or how a person could increase the doses with much less adjusting than it required when lowering the dose. I have spent many nights working up great distractions.

Whenever I was able to feel truly okay on the new dose by the end of seven days I figured that I was doing great. When it took fourteen or fifteen days I struggled with discouragement. I really needed my cheerleader Necia and our kids' help. They never judged me, condemned me for taking morphine but they were all pleased when I stopped taking morphine.

Discouragement comes easily -
Once I made the commitment to get off of morphine I had to guard against feelings of shame. I truly did feel very guilty. Maybe not guilty but something strong and negative. I found myself in a frame of mind, once or twice, to think dumb thoughts like "why try, I am weak so why try?" What a nightmare this little adventure could be.

Over the years several people had told me that I would rue the day I started taking morphine because there was no way out. I always argued, at least in my mind, that there had to be. I had no idea how difficult it would be. It was back to that same two-edged sword i.e. finding balance. When increasing the dose it was trying to manage the pain so that I could live life with some semblance of intelligence.

The goal was to not be crazy from pain and not be crazy from drug-induced stupidity. Reducing doses was also like playing with a two-edged sword. Trying to take away some of the drug stupidity without allowing the pain to consume me.

It seems to me that the greatest temptation in the entire affair was to not allow oneself to become completely self-centered. Both sides of the sword were all about me. I had to somehow focus enough to be successful and sometimes that took a long time and completely consumed me with trying to strike that balance. How can a person do that and not become selfish, turned in?

Less selfishness -

The answer was not completely new; it was an extension of the old distraction game but much more rewarding. I usually had to do the distraction game much the same as always. To this I added a distraction of service. How can I sit on the love seat and occupy myself with some problem or book or YouTube lecture or documentary when my sweetheart was not well and she slaved away all the time taking care of me? Simple, I would help her. So, much like a little boy who is inspired by the Sunday School lesson on Mother's Day I set about to do the best I could.

About this time my Paget's was really in full bloom. The pain was there sure enough but with it came intense feelings of terrible sickness. I struggled to find something I could do to make a difference.

The answers should not have eluded me or thought by me to be difficult. I could load the dishwasher by myself. I could unload it by myself. I could wash whatever needs to be washed by hand. I could ask her what I could do whenever something needs to be done. I could slice the fruit, the cheese and the vegetables and help prepare the meals. I could operate the clothes washing machine and the dryer...sometimes I had to ask instructions but then I could do stuff while she was resting. I could fold the clothes when doing the laundry. I could even run the carpet cleaner to spot clean where the cat had harfed up her last hairball. I cleaned the cat's litter box every night. Seeing how much time these things saved her really has rewarded me. Her thanks and appreciation are the kindest I know. But the real reward is seeing her not have to labor so as she struggles with her own pain. It was getting hard for her to be on her feet and I could make a big difference there. So I was rewarded with me not thinking only of myself and by seeing her burdens lifted a little bit.

It gets harder as doses drop -

The second adjustment was much like the first; one dose took two weeks and the other two daily doses took only one week each. Again, this took a total of four weeks. So, I had dropped all three daily doses by 30mg in a two month period. That sounded good to me for as long as I did not think about the reductions ahead. Still, I was more than half way to complete freedom from morphine. I still had to stop using 62.5 mg per day to complete this journey.

The second round of reductions was harder than the first. It seemed that it took four or five days for my body to adjust to the point that I was not lying awake in pain. The withdrawals were more severe on the second round. Pain was my constant companion and the pain grew more severe with each reduction in dose. Even with all of the good I could already see happening when I was on reduced doses the old hag was back with her siren-song promising me pleasure, relief and freedom from the unending pain.

I felt that my up-front resolve was sufficient to see me through the entire process of getting this great burden out of my life. I found myself fighting both the pain and the addiction and had to renew that resolve with each reduction in dose. Without a doubt each renewal was more demanding, more reality-based than the one before. I was dealing with more pain and the withdrawal symptoms were more severe. My resolve had to be greater and my integrity with my resolve had to be more secure. There was no room for cheating. By the time I was half way through the process I was able to see that any cheating would cost me more personal suffering in the long run. And it would cost my family and friends who were trying so very hard to support me and put up with me as I was going through my struggles.

This was another example of how the hag would try to break my commitment. Guilt. Guilt would be a part of every detail of this journey. Guilt for ever becoming addicted; guilt for having tried and failed a couple of times; guilt for feeling so tempted to stay on a certain dose longer (happened with every reduction in every dose); guilt for wanting to ask to go back to a previously higher dose; guilt for getting so sick, guilt for every symptom of withdrawal; guilt for all the time and attention needed to coach me, cheer me, express confidence in me; guilt for being an addict...guilt for feeling guilty. I still struggle with all of the guilt. 15 years of my life given to the hag!

The third round of reductions was much more difficult than either of the first two. I thought that it would get easier as I took less and less. It was much more difficult with each successive round of reductions. I don't know whether it would have made a difference to me to have known how much more difficult each step down in medication would be. Once there the fear/realization that if I went backwards I would have to cover ground already gained again if I was to ever break free of the old hag – that helped me to keep trying to move forward from where I had gotten to. If I had known how difficult it would be before I arrived there would I have even made it to that point? I want to believe that I would have always kept my resolve, always kept trying, always spit in the eye of the hag and moved forward. Would I have done so? I know I would not have done so without the help I received from my faith, my sweetheart, my family and friends. My grandchildren's influences was a terrific help.

Who/what is controlling who/what?

I remembered that as a kid I had a neighbor living a couple of blocks away who drank alcohol much of the time. I had, rather arrogantly (self righteously?), thought on multiple occasions that he should just stop drinking so he didn't do embarrassing stuff. Now I had a question: Did he continue to drink because he liked to drink or did he continue to drink so he didn't have to go through withdrawals? I could see how answering that question either way would be logical, believable, and understandable from my newly acquired viewpoint. I also thought of another question: Why did people call it substance abuse? The substance, whatever it was, probably couldn't even feel, certainly did not think. I was not abusing the substance; the substance was abusing me. I would add thinking about how I could quit being so harsh in my judgment of other people to my list of distractions. That thought could command a lot of time that I was otherwise wasting as I tried to get off of morphine.

This thought called to my remembrance a little song my grandfather used to sing to us grandkids. The song was about a fellow who had gone hunting for bear. It was unclear to me whether the bear found him or if he found the bear. But a great contest began. The bear was chasing the hunter who observed that the bear was gaining on him as he tried to escape the event. The hunter decided that his best, maybe only, option was to pray. So the man began to call out in prayer asking the Lord to help him. The final words of his prayer (and the song) was "please Lord, if you don't help me, don't help that darn bear."

Morphine (the old hag in this booklet) must not have help. As we pray for God to not help the old hag we must pray for his help for the addict. And we must do more than pray; we must listen, help, encourage, cheer and love. I believe that every recovering addict must be running as fast as they can to get away from the old hag. And so they go around and around and around...and around. There can be only one winner and the price is beyond counting if the old hag wins.

And it gets harder still; more D Ts -

On the third round of reduction my nose ran almost constantly whenever it had been more than a few hours since a dose. It was terrible. I could type an entire page of this booklet and in that time I could wet almost all of a paper towel from the discharge from my nose. I had that crawling, panicking feeling much of the time. It was there much of the time but the intensity was less. So even though I was sweating profusely and nasal discharge was nearly always active, I considered that to be a huge improvement.

Believe it or not, the running nose was an extreme frustration in part because it interfered with me helping my sweetheart do stuff. It would not be sanitary to unload the dishwasher and put the contents into their proper cabinets, drawers, etc. when one's nose is dripping, dripping, dripping. On a few occasions I tore pieces of the paper towel off and used them to just plug my nose completely then wash my hands again and proceed to help. Whenever I was helping by doing things that made me walk around the kitchen, load the washer/dryer and go fetch stuff from the basement or the fridge in the garage all gave me the opportunity to move about in a structured, purposeful way so I did not have to just stand in place and dance the D T dance. This all worked out well. This was a very good thing. Thinking of her rather than brooding over my problems was one of the healthiest things I have ever done. I hope I have the health to do this as long as I live. Perhaps just as important, I hope I remember the lesson and do not allow selfishness to find its way between us. It really felt good to look outward for opportunities.

It will never surprise anyone who knows Necia to learn that she has been grateful for every little thing I have ever done to help her. She regularly inquires about how I am feeling, what I am thinking about things. She always validates with me whether I am feeling well enough to do the little things I do for her.

She regularly inquired about whether I was needing medicine for breakthrough pain or if I was reducing too fast, etc. She frequently assured me that she would give me whatever doses I required. All I needed to do was tell her I needed it. This has been an important part of my quitting morphine. Although we keep all of our prescription drugs in a locked safe to which she has the only key. That was not a trust issue, it was a mental issue and a security issue.

Sometimes I confused things, which I believe to be an artifact of the Paget's disease and/or an artifact of the morphine. She has kept a written record of every dose of every prescription for years. She would have given me the key if I had only asked and all that she would have asked in return was that I made sure by double checking with her that the dose I was going to take was what I was wanting to take and that it was a safe dose. If I was having a difficult day she would offer to get things (medicines and/or different supplements) for me. Having the safe locked forced me to not give in to a moment of panic or other withdrawal symptoms just because I had to formulate in words to tell why I wanted the key. Along side that was her promise that she would support me in any way I wanted. If I needed more morphine I could have had it without any discussion beyond what was necessary to establish that I was not doing something that was reckless or unsafe. This has been a very important component to me succeeding in this effort to be free from morphine. I believe I have asked her for a half-tablet of the immediate release morphine perhaps a couple of dozen times in 15 years.

This is really difficult; Necia asserts herself-

Round four consists of removing the IR (immediate release) stuff. I saved this for last because if we had to cut them into smaller doses and take them closer together to keep the level of morphine in my blood level, that could easily be done. It would be dangerous to cut the extended release pills because it would likely release the morphine into my body much faster than desirable or healthy. The coating on the extended release pills limits how fast the morphine is released. If someone cuts those pills with a pill cutter the integrity of the timed release would be completely compromised.

The little guys are the most difficult -

Eliminating the last (7.5mg) doses were the most difficult. If a dose was late I would go into D Ts within a couple of hours. Sometimes I would have DT-light the entire time between doses. I would have all of the symptoms of full-blown D Ts but at a reduced intensity. It was very difficult but doable. Yes, this was extremely difficult business. It seemed impossible more than a few times.

When we removed the last of the 15mg extended release tablets I was confident that I was amazing, wonderful...etc. After two days on just the immediate release pills at 7.5mg I told Necia that I wanted her to skip one of my doses. Her reply didn't shock me but it made me think. She told me that I was still running in place in bed every night all night long ...from removing the last extended release tablet. Based on this I told her that I needed to stay at a 3x/day schedule on 7.5 mg. I was so worn out from the shock and trauma of removing that last extended release dose that I was pleading for help. She took control and said that we were not going to lose our discipline; we are going to take away the remaining doses by cutting the 7.5mg doses in half and take them every 4 hours then remove the doses one by one, after a week or two. I must admit (again) that I hate the D Ts – all of the symptoms of quitting.

I certainly needed a solid helping hand at this point. It seemed almost as if just the mentioning of taking any morphine away from me would kill me. I was in the D Ts at some level for almost a week. I just could not get that desperate need out of my mind. This actually happened at some level three times over about five weeks. I say mind but it was much more physical than mental. At this time it would be a toss-up between the D Ts and pain. Having taken so much morphine away the pain from Paget's disease, as well as the car wreck injury, were screaming nearly every minute. Maybe I was going to go nuts from both. If so I hoped that the fact there were two reasons for my struggle perhaps it would only take half as long to complete this goal of being morphine free before the end of June. It ended up taking about five and a half months for me to get clean of morphine with much struggling for all that time.

As it turned out the new brand of legal, hemp-derived CBD oil with the two additives taken with the anxiety relief tablets provided me with a lot of pain reduction. Sometimes it seemed to be close to what the morphine had done. Other times it seemed that it was much like the morphine and it seemed like it was not doing anything at all. Then, in the very last couple of weeks Necia identified three essential oils with excellent pain reducing characteristics...just a few drops of each per day. I believe I may not have to ask my doctor for any kind of substitute drugs! I would just put one drop, two or three if I was in elevated levels of pain, in the glass I filled with water to take my pills with.

It has been very educational doing this little project. I don't think I could be successful if I was relying just on my good intentions as I reduced dosing. I doubt I could have maintained a consistent dose if I was just going to use pure willpower. I needed help; I needed a process; I needed support. My process has been a schedule and distractions, especially prayer and more distraction. When my head was hurting bad and I was not sleeping because of pain and I was beginning to grouch I needed a way to put my mind to work doing something that had some level of demand and it had to distract me from even thinking about drugs. This fact, I believe, makes it very important to choose distractions that truly interest the person escaping addiction. Any old topic is too flimsy to embrace the intense distraction required.

My distractions that I have shared in this booklet are not magic and they may not work for anyone else. I used many, many more than are on the list in this booklet. But as I said earlier, other people in severe pain have told me that distractions were helpful to them. Everyone is different which means that everyone will almost certainly need to make at least a part of their own list of methods and of distractions. Borrowing them from someone else is a wonderful thing to do if they will work for you.

Perhaps legal, hemp-derived CBD oil and other natural things may help you. They continue to help me in a big way. (18 months and counting!) Will the day come that I need something prescribed? That is possible, more likely the longer I live, as my condition worsens. But I promise you all that if I am conscious I will do my best to never again take morphine.

I must not forget to give special mention to my latest distraction of looking outward to see if there are things I can do for my sweetheart. They are the best. Getting outside of myself, getting past at least some of the selfishness has been the thing that facilitated getting off of those last small doses, which were the most difficult steps.

A final statement of fact...

While I was taking morphine I was very seldom free from pain. It is also true that I sometimes wondered if the morphine was doing anything at all because the pain level was so high. My experience with the natural remedies has netted very nearly the same results; sometimes I was (am) at level one – little or no pain; sometimes the pain would (will) prevent me from sleeping for 36 hours or more. The pattern is very similar; one or two days per month (occasionally up to four) I am awake for 36 hours, or more, because of pain. A huge difference is that the morphine carries with it such an arsenal of side effects and is so intrusive to living with any degree of personal freedom that even if the pain was a little worse on the natural stuff that is the way I would go every time.

This booklet was written with the hope that others might find some help getting off of drugs. Hopefully it may help others to stay off of drugs. I have been brutally honest; invited you into my emotions, my fears, my weaknesses, my suicidal thoughts, even shared my health problems. More than all this I have shared very private moments as Necia has helped me. This could be really embarrassing stuff if some people with some attitudes read it. I have decided that that is okay if it helps someone.

I hope you will realize that you have walked on sacred ground. I ask that as you meet others who are trapped in an opiate world that you tread lightly and do not leave tracks in their sacred ground. Not just the deliberate abuser but the persons who are in serious pain and have somehow gotten themselves addicted and reliant on drugs to a point that is not good. I know that a person can become suicidal when they are taking a lot of morphine (or other drugs) and they may feel that it has stolen their life. You can kick it, especially if you have a little help. And help is waiting.

A loved one, perhaps the significant other, if a person has that relationship, can be very helpful... if you have the commitment. That loved one, and it can be your cat or your dog or your canary...will be trusting you to get yourself arranged so that you can do what you want to do for them to sweeten their lives WITH YOU. I agree with the Alcoholics Anonymous folks that a belief in a higher/greater power is helpful and enabling in ways that nothing else can be.

In nearly all communities there are free addiction recovery programs sponsored by churches, civic groups, hospitals, neighborhoods, etc. If they understand exactly what it is you need them to help you do there are very few who would not be happy to help you without judgment or accusation of any kind. (I know some of them in my church.) When someone asks for help the amount of compassion shown may surprise just about everyone. The people staffing recovery programs may have to *act* 'tough' sometimes but love abounds.

Addiction recovery is a hellish experience – or can be. Traveling that path alone is a very difficult journey – it may have been impossible for me. It is a difficult journey if you have good company and a lot of support. I know this; I am not just parroting something I heard someone say or something I read in a book. I just completed the journey and although it has been very difficult it is very much something a person can do with support. It took me five and a half months to get clean and in all that time I was treated with only love and kindness. No exceptions except the one ER doctor!

I have never tasted alcohol, never smoked tobacco or pot and never taken an illegal drug. I have never abused a prescription drug. But, I have had a prescription drug abuse me. My heartfelt thanks to God, to my primary care physician, the pain clinic and to my sweetheart, my family and my cat Katie; I am morphine free for 17 1/2 months (I keep saying 18 months-yes I am proud) as this booklet is uploaded for printing! That is a really big deal!

And *that* is worth all the effort and distractions. And now? It is time for me to get back to living life; hoping to find more of those buried memories along the way!

What are you going to do?

****Please note** that it was deliberate that no product names or caregiver names, beside my wife Necia, my family and my cat were mentioned anywhere in this booklet because I cannot prescribe and I do not want anyone to think this booklet is an advertisement or an endorsement. Besides, even with help you still have to do the work; all the heavy lifting. The point is you CAN do it and at least one person (me) has found help from nature!